A DOCTOR'S LINE

Also by this author

A DOCTOR'S LINE

Poetry and Prescriptions in Health and Healing

Kenneth C. Calman

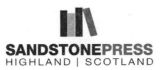

SANDSTONEPRESS
HIGHLAND | SCOTLAND

First published in Great Britain
and the USA in 2014 by
Sandstone Press Ltd
Scottish Provincial Press Building
Dochcarty Road
Dingwall
Ross-shire
IV15 9UG
Scotland.

www.sandstonepress.com

The publisher acknowledges support from
Creative Scotland towards publication of this volume.

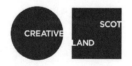

ISBN: 978-1-908737-89-2
ISBNe: 978-1-908737-91-5

Cover design by Mark Ecob
Typesetting by Iolaire Typesetting, Newtonmore
Printed and bound by Ozgraf, Poland

Contents

Preface

This book tells the story of health and medicine in Scotland over a period of 700 years through the medium of Scotland's literature. *Makars and Mediciners,* the original title, began as a personal commonplace book, an anthology, of novels, poems and short stories, which linked Scottish literature and medicine. This, in itself, grew out of a short course on literature and medicine for medical students as part of the course on medical ethics at the University of Glasgow (1984–1989); the importance of literature and the arts in general, in professional education and in improving health and well-being, was emphasised. These interests expanded in the University of Durham with the establishment of a Centre for the Arts and Humanities in Health and Medicine. In this Centre, the impact of the arts and humanities on health is being explored in the growing field of Medical Humanities. One of the objectives of this book is to make Scottish literature on health and medicine readily accessible to a wide audience of both health professionals and the public. The theme of the commonplace book will be developed during the course of this volume.

There are a number of ways and levels in which the literature of any country or genre may be explored; through its language, realism, historical accuracy, and many others. In this book the literature of Scotland is explored in two ways. First how the literature illuminates and illustrates issues of health and medicine; and secondly, and perhaps more importantly, how these can be used to assist in learning, particularly of medical students and doctors, but also of the wider public. This examination is not based on a critical study of the literature in formal terms, but through literature, it records the medical, cultural, historical and social changes over 700 years.

My purpose has been to provide a resource for those interested in improving health and in changing clinical practice: for debate, discussion, agreement and disagreement, learning, and to stimulate a broader interest in the role the arts can play. Ultimately its purpose is to show some of the ways in which a study of literature can be used to fuel debate about the improvement of health and health care. It is hoped that some of the readings, by demonstrating experience of issues of the past, and of the present, will be of sufficient power to change thinking and practice. The power of the word is significant and can change attitudes and behaviour. The book should also be relevant to the general public, patients and carers, as they consider consequences of a particular issue of health, illness, diagnosis or treatment.

Inevitably, the choice of extracts is restricted and they represent my personal readings and preferences. The reader may well have more to add. As will be noted later in the book, Sir William Olser, a very distinguished medical writer, notes that his textbook of medicine was to bring him 'mind to mind' with the reader. Perhaps this book will do the same.

Acknowledgements

It is my pleasure to record my thanks to Professor Gerard Carruthers and Professor Kirsteen McCue for their unfailing support. Their help has been invaluable. I particularly wish to mention the role of Professor Robin Downie in its genesis. He was a special mentor when I needed it most and a good friend. I should also like to thank colleagues from the School of Critical Studies at the University of Glasgow, particularly Professor Alan Riach, for their input into the project. I would also like to thank Professor Jane MacNaughton and her colleagues at the Centre for Arts and Humanities in Health and Medicine at the University of Durham for her encouragement and support. My thanks also go to Dr. Linden Bicket for her help in formatting and referencing the work and Sheila Kidd for her help with the Gaelic translations. Hugh Cheape from Sabhal Mòr Ostaig on Skye was always helpful. Other members of staff across the University have been very supportive and encouraged me to finish the work.

Libraries have been at the heart of this research and I am grateful to the University of Glasgow Library and its Archives, the Mitchell Library in Glasgow, the National Library of Scotland, the British Library, the Library of the Royal Society of Medicine, Innerpeffray Library Perthshire and the British Medical Association Library in London. I should particularly like to thank Knightswood Public Library, a small community library in a housing estate in the west of Glasgow, where in the 1940s and 1950s I spent much time as a boy reading and thinking. Such local libraries remain an essential part of the community though their function has continually developed and changed. I should also like to thank my school teachers in both primary and secondary education, though now a very long time ago, who contributed greatly to my understanding and love of books.

It is a pleasure to thank the staff of Sandstone Press for their help and encouragement, and in particular to Moira Forsyth for her encouragement and attention to detail.

In this book there are many quotations from authors and books both well-known and less well known. These are respectfully and gratefully made under the accepted principle of fair dealing, and references are contained within the text of this book and its notes. Three who are quoted in excess of the accepted norm are Janice Galloway, Hugh MacDiarmid, and Edwin Morgan. To them, their successors, and their publishers I give particular thanks in addition to the prescribed words following:-

A lengthy extract in Chapter Sixteen from *Janice Galloway* by *THE TRICK IS TO KEEP BREATHING*. Published by *Vintage*. Reprinted by permission of The Random House Group Limited.

Various extracts from *Hugh MacDiarmid COMPLETE POEMS* Volume One (1993), Edited by Michael Grieve and W. R. Aitken, published by Carcanet Press Limited.

'Gorgo and Beau' is quoted in full from A BOOK OF LIVES by Edwin Morgan (2007), published by Carcanet Press Limited.

I am also grateful to my wife and family for allowing me to do this and for their encouragement and positive criticism, and to my new granddaughter Grace who diverted my attention to another range of writings. Finally I should like to thank my dog Mungo who started me on this project and my new puppy Ailsa who has continued to give me time to think as we had our walks and make notes in my wee book.

CHAPTER 1

Setting the scene

Introduction

Health is increasingly important to all of us, as is the care provided to patients and their families by the members of the health-care team. In this book a history of the changes in practice and understanding of clinical care and public health in Scotland will be considered using the literature of Scotland. It will explore these matters as expressed by writers and poets to illustrate just how much has changed. The readings will, hopefully, allow discussion and debate on a wide range of topics.

The purpose of this book, therefore, is to review the possibility that a study of the literature of Scotland could contribute to a better understanding of the changing role of the doctor, the values of the medical profession and how the health of the population might be improved. This introductory chapter, and the questions which are set out in it, will be re-considered at the end of the book, as part of the continuing debate.

This book grew out of a series of learning experiences presented to medical students during the ethics class in the Faculty of Medicine in the University of Glasgow in the 1980s, in association with Professor Robin Downie from the Department of Moral Philosophy. We began to introduce fragments of novels and poetry to illustrate aspects of medical practice and this grew into a small voluntary class entitled 'Literature and Medicine'.[1] With this as a basis I expanded this interest, focussing on Scottish literature, but with the same overall purpose; to better understand the role of the profession of medicine, its value base and the link between the humanities and science, relating particularly to the period between the 14th century and the present. In this context I was delighted to learn of the publication of a short book of poems for new medical graduates (*Tools of the Trade: Poems for new doctors*, Edinburgh, Scottish Poetry Library,

1

2014) which aims to provide doctors with supportive and encouraging literature.

Just as the medical profession has changed over the last 700 years, so Scotland has also changed dramatically. Since the time when our story begins, Scotland's population, demography, constitution, industrial base, education and literature have altered, as with many other places in the western world, out of all recognition. External events such as the Reformation, the French and American Revolutions and a series of world wars, have also had a significant impact on Scotland. The population of Scotland, for example, has grown from around 600,000 at the beginning of the 18th century to over five million at the start of the 21st century.[2] The age structure of the population has also significantly changed, becoming more elderly, and there has been a rise in urban populations often centred near major industries.

Changes to health and medicine over this period are no exception. Life span has increased, treatment and care have been improved, the role of doctors has been re-defined, new diseases have appeared – and old ones disappeared, attitudes to life and death have changed and public understanding of health and illness radically modified. In other words, the world of health and human circumstance in Scotland, as elsewhere, is a story that continues to unfold.

The particular issue for consideration in this book is how the literature of Scotland reflects these changes and what pointers it gives to the understanding of illness and disease. In addition it will consider how the role of the doctor has changed and what the influence has been of the scientific basis of medicine and health on Scottish literature. As patterns of illness have changed so the doctor has become more active and interventionist but is also judged more critically on what she or he has achieved. As one example of this, childhood mortality, mainly related to infectious disease, has been reduced significantly. Smallpox, often referred to in the earlier literature, has now been eradicated worldwide. In a similar way a walk through any 19th century cemetery or burial ground will show the extent of childhood mortality with, in many cases, four or five children dying in the same family group, something very rarely seen at the start of the 21st century. Violence, on the other hand, was a significant cause of death in the earlier centuries and remains so today.[3]

This subject is therefore approached from a particular perspective and clinical tradition: it began with an interest in ethics, and has continued with a broader involvement in storytelling, imagination, feeling and sentiment in further defining the evidence base, and in clarifying the process of learning of doctors over the centuries.[4] Its origin was also based on a commonplace book, kept by myself, of poems, books, quotations which were of interest, and which stimulated new thinking and approaches. It is also concerned about the future of medical and health care practice, and what can be learned from the arts.

This raises a more fundamental issue, that of the purpose of the arts. Murray Pittock makes the point clearly and indicates the ways in which this book will engage:

What then are the arts for? Pursued as they should be, they serve to provide the context to evaluate claims of novelty, to frame policy and prevent us from doing the same thing twice; to understand persuasion, propaganda and the language of the situation and negotiate it, to console and heal; to empower and provide the space in which we can be, and communicate that on every level.[5]

The wider background

There are at least four dimensions which can be identified when considering changes in health and health care and which need some background to enable a consideration of the readings which follow; the health of the public and communities, the care of the individual, the science and understanding of health and disease and the ethics and value base of the profession of medicine. These interact and find a focus in the quality of life for individuals and communities and the professional characteristics of the doctor and other clinical professionals. The professional dimension will be considered in the following chapter.

Health and its determinants

A definition of health

The World Health Organisation's (WHO) definition of health is a good starting point. It states that health 'is a state of complete physical and mental well-being and not merely the absence of disease or infirmity'.[6] Several issues follow from this definition. First, that health is a relative term and cannot be regarded as an absolute, in that it can always be improved. Second, there are both positive and negative aspects of health. Feeling well and being ill are both part of the same concept. Finally, health should be regarded in an holistic way, in that many factors are relevant; physical, emotional, spiritual, psychological, social and intellectual (the PEPSI concept).

The determinants of health

To assist in the process of identifying aspects of Scottish literature that might be relevant, it is useful to provide a framework within which to gather material that illuminates issues related to health and medicine. One such framework is to consider the range of factors that determine health.

Five broad categories can be identified as determining the health of an individual or population. For each of these categories, descriptions can be found in the literature of Scotland and the insights provided by the authors can add significantly to our understanding of the public's response to health messages and changes in health. The generally accepted determinants are briefly described as follows.

Social and economic factors   Influences such as employment, education and financial circumstances all have a major impact on health. In a city such as Glasgow moving from one street to another in the same part of town can see significant differences in health. The health effects of poverty and deprivation are well recorded in the medical literature. The rapid development of Glasgow as a major urban centre in the 19th century, with little infrastructure at this stage and little social support, demonstrates how quickly the effects of deprivation can be seen and related to poor health. Novels about Glasgow in the 20th century illustrate these effects clearly.

Lifestyle   Related to social and economic issues is the lifestyle that individuals or communities adopt and that are chosen by them. These include very well-known factors such as lack of exercise, obesity, cigarette smoking, drugs and alcohol abuse. Some of these relate to social and economic factors but are independent of them. Other examples of this are the sexually transmitted diseases which feature in many poems and novels. The clinical descriptions of syphilis, for example, in 18th century literature make it clear that the diagnosis was readily recognised. By the 20th century novels such as *Trainspotting* by Irving Welsh (1993) set out in graphic detail the current range of lifestyle issues such as drug abuse that affect health.

The environment   Environmental issues play an important part in influencing health. These include such issues as housing, air and water quality, and the transmission of infection. The descriptions in books, plays and poems of the living conditions of the people of Scotland provide an invaluable source of information on the details of family life and living. A particularly good example of how health, medicine and housing interact was seen in the appointment of Scotland's first Medical Officer of Health in Edinburgh. At 1.00am on the morning of Sunday 24th November 1861 the tenement at 99–103 High Street collapsed with a huge noise and thirty-five people were killed. This was Paisley's Close, and during the rescue operation a boy who was trapped shouted to his rescuers 'Heave awa lads I'm no deid yet' and he was eventually rescued. His head – and his comments with lads changed to 'chaps' – remain carved on the lintel of the close to this day. There was such an outcry from the public that an Officer of Health was appointed, Dr Henry Duncan Littlejohn (later Sir Henry) (1826–1914) to take things forward. In his application for the post he was supported by Sir James Young Simpson (1811–1870) and Professor James Syme (1799–1870), two of the leading medical men in Edinburgh at the time. Thus began the formal link between health and social and environmental issues.[7]

Health services   Over the period of study this aspect of health has also changed hugely. From a medically-based service in the 14th to mid-20th century with some nurse and midwife support and itinerant healers, to a modern day health service, multi-disciplinary and strongly evidence-based. From an essentially home based service, to one which is institutionally based and technology driven.

At the beginning of our story there were few doctors and a limited number of hospitals. Care was often provided by local healers or midwives, through the use of manuals such as Buchan's *Domestic Medicine*, or was more generally self-care. There was no state provision and it was not until 1948 that this became available. Folk cures were the norm and were encouraged (Fergusson's 'Caller Oysters' (1772) described in chapter seven, fits into this category) and many households kept a medicine bottle to deal with all eventualities. In the *Wee MacGreegor* stories by J.J. Bell (1933) for example there is always a bottle of 'Ile' (castor oil) available to deal with the effects of eating too many sweeties.

Mental health issues have been dealt with in a variety of ways over the centuries and again are reflected in the literature. These are to be found in the descriptions of mental illness in such books as the *Memoirs of a Justified Sinner* (1824), and *Dr Jekyll and Mr Hyde* (1886) through to Janice Galloway's treatment of anorexia in *The Trick is to Keep Breathing* (1999).

The rise of institutional places of care has been one of the most significant aspects of the development of health services. These 'Castles of Healing' have become dominant in modern health care and a far cry from the single handed 'good doctor' in the 'Kailyard' literature.

Genetics and basic biological mechanisms of disease Over the 700 year period under review our understanding of health and disease has increased enormously. From initial discoveries in anatomy, physiology and pathology, through to the determination of the human genome, each of the developments has taken us a step closer to controlling illness and improving health. The identification of infectious agents and the pathology of disease have made major contributions to this. Much of our health is pre-determined by our genes, but much can be done to modify the possible consequences by an understanding of the other determinants of health.

There are, of course, significant interactions between each of these determinants. They are all related, and the determination of health is multi-factorial. For example the provision of health care in a rural environment can, and may, mean some compromises in the range of services immediately available. Other examples would include the link between obesity and the morbidity from surgical operations and the relationship between lifestyle, deprivation and health.

Nevertheless it is generally possible to identify, in particular individuals and populations, factors which are especially important. One aspect which flows from this is the potential for good health if the factors which we already know about were taken seriously by you and me and in communities across the country. Some time ago I published a book with the title *The Potential for Health*[8] which argued that if we took the current advice on smoking, exercise, diet, alcohol and drugs, we would all be much healthier. The question, which will come up again and again, is why we still ignore the advice. In another book, written a few years later, I proposed a 'contagious theory of behaviour change'[9] in which I suggested that stories and the arts could be used to change attitudes and behaviour. This is one aspect of this book which will be followed up later.

Quality of life

Quality of life is difficult to measure or even to define. Clearly quality of life can only be described and measured in individual terms, and depends on present lifestyle, past experience, hopes for the future, dreams and ambitions. Quality of life must include all areas of life and experience and take into account the impact of illness and treatment. A good quality of life may be said to be present when the hopes of an individual are matched and fulfilled by experience. The opposite can be said to be true – a poor quality of life occurs when hopes do not meet with experience.[10]

Quality of life changes with time and under normal circumstances can vary considerably. The priorities and goals of an individual must be realistic and would therefore be expected to change with time and be modified by age and experience. To improve quality of life therefore it is necessary to try to narrow the gap between the hopes and aspirations, and what actually happens. The aim is to help people reach the goals they have set for themselves, or to reduce their expectations. A good quality of life is usually expressed in terms of contentment, satisfaction, happiness, fulfilment, and the ability to cope.

From this definition of quality of life certain implications follow, namely that:

• It can only be assessed and described by the individual – what I mean by quality of life may be different from your concept. It must take into account many aspects of life and must be related to individual goals and aspirations which should be realistic.

- Improvement is related to the ability to identify and achieve these goals and illness and treatment may well modify these goals. The gap between expectation and reality may be the driving force for some individuals.

- Action may be required to narrow the potential gap. This action may be taken by the patient alone or with the help of others. As each goal is achieved new ones are identified opening up the gap once again. It is a constantly changing picture.

Quality of life therefore measures the difference at a particular moment between the hopes and expectations of the individual and the individual's present experiences. Quality of life has many dimensions covering all life areas including home and garden, work, hobbies, family, financial issues, body image, diet, mobility, ambitions, spiritual issues and concepts of the future. Part of the role of the doctor in caring for patients is thus to assist in improving quality of life. It is possible to be healthy and have a poor quality of life, and even in poor health, quality of life can be maintained.

Death too has a particular importance in the literature of Scotland, and is relevant to quality of life. From the 'Lament for the Makaris' by William Dunbar in the 15th century and its recurring line 'Timor mortis conturbat me' (The fear of death disturbs me) to the 'Dying words of Bonny Heck' in the 18th century and the 'Elegies' of Douglas Dunn, in the 20th century, death has been a constant theme, and will be considered in this review.

Within the many novels and poems to be considered in this book there are numerous examples of what quality of life was like in Scotland over the generations. These add depth and colour to the impact of methods of changing health and treating illness.

A critical approach to the literature of Scotland in relation to health and medicine

Literary criticism involves making judgements on the writings of an author, a work or a genre; but judgement in relation to what? Should it be enjoyment, popularity of the work or author, morality, seriousness, realism or personal and professional background? Or should it be in relation to a particular perspective: feminism, national culture, gay issues, ecology etc. There is generally a requirement for a close reading or analysis of the text. Fashions, of course, change in literature and an author such as Walter Scott had huge popularity and high critical acclaim in the 19th century, but less so now, although the *New Edinburgh Edition of the Waverley Novels* (2000–9) has sold over 100,000 copies and there is a new generation of Scott scholars. On the other hand some aspects of literature, such as the 'Kailyard School', were not well received when first published, but have recently been re-evaluated.[11] In addition the criticism must take into account the time of writing, the context (e.g. the knowledge of science and disease) the place and setting of the work.

In this volume, the judgements on the authors and passages chosen, relate to the ability of the text (or in most instances a short section of the text) to illustrate particular aspects of health, medicine or the work of the doctor. For this reason these readings have been chosen to stimulate thinking either of the reader or of groups of people in teaching or learning environments, book clubs or patients groups.

A wide range of authors has been chosen to illustrate the thoughts and discussion in the book and the selection has been to allow as much depth as possible. The possible range is enormous from the 'classics' (Burns and Scott etc.) to the popular *(Wee MacGreegor)*. It is hoped that these extracts will reflect how Scottish literature has helped to shape thinking on health and medicine. The book can be read from cover to cover, or dipped into for topics of particular interest.

Four examples are chosen here to illustrate the principles of this approach and each will be followed up further in the appropriate section of the book.

Robert Henryson

Henryson (1420–1490) was one of the great mediaeval makars. In his poem 'The Abbey Walk' he identifies some of the spirit of the times, the religious ethos and the lack of effective therapy and medical skill.

Thoch thou be blind, or have ane halt [limp]
Or in thy face deformit ill,
Sae it come nocht throu thy default
No man suld thee reprief by skill [reprove]
Blame nocht thy Lord, sae is his will;
Spurn nocht thy fute againis the wall;
But with meek hairt and prayer still
Obey and thank thy God of all[12]

The tone is negative and submissive, and is in accord with the times.

Robert Burns

In the 'Address to the unco guid, or the rigidly righteous', Burns sets out a very modern view of the problems of developing a habit of drinking to excess.

See Social Life and Glee sit down
All joyous and unthinking,
Till, quite transmugrify'd, they're grown
Debauchery and drinking:
O, would they stay to calculate
Th' eternal consequences,
Or your more dreaded hell to state-
Damnation of expenses![13]

Is it as simple as that? Do we just sit down and have a good time with friends and slowly sink into debauchery? Is this the only way in which bad, or unhealthy behaviours start? How can unhealthy behaviour be changed?

Dr John Brown

One of the most interesting of the short stories by Dr John Brown (1810–1882) is entitled 'Rab and his friends'.[14] Further reference will be made to this later, but it is a story of a medical student in Edinburgh in the days before anaesthetics. Rab is a dog who accompanies James, a carrier, everywhere and indeed comes into the operating theatre. The patient, Ailie is married to James, and she is obviously suffering from cancer of the breast. She has her first discussion with the doctor, as the narrator, a medical student, tells us:

> Next day, my master, the surgeon, examined Ailie. There was no doubt it must kill her, and soon. It could be removed – it might never return – it would give her speedy relief – she should have it done. She curtsied, looked at James, and said, 'When?' 'Tomorrow', said the kind surgeon – a man of few words. She and James and Rab and I retired. I noticed that he and she spoke little, but seemed to anticipate everything in each other.[15]

There are two possible views on this conversation. The first is that such was the trust between the doctor and the patient that little in the way of information exchange was necessary. The second is that such communication is woefully inadequate. Almost no information on possible side effects, length of stay and long-term consequences is discussed with Ailie. These two views are as relevant today as they were then, and they are still debated.

William McIlvanney

McIlvanney's (b. 1936) novel *Docherty* looks at life in a shipyard community, struggling with the problems of the Depression, unemployment, and living standards. At the very beginning of the book Tam Docherty is born, and the words of the doctor who delivers him are worth recording.

> The laughter ebbed to a still contentment. . . . Dr Allan leaned into the cushion of heat behind him. His professionalism being disarmed by tiredness, he saw the scene as a fortress of people built protectively and perhaps hopelessly round a child. He remembered how at the birth he had put the child to the bottom of the bed, a parcel of useless flesh, while he concerned himself with the mother. It was Mrs Ritchie who had skelped him into life. She would talk about that and it would swell in the telling, would become a story of a life stolen from the jaws of death. . . . As the doctor lifted the glass again to his mouth, it was a private toast. With it there went a solemn wish for the kind of fulfilment to this beginning that they dreamt of. It was wished for all the more intensely because he could not for a second begin to believe in it.[16]

Here is an exhausted but happy doctor, described after the delivery of Docherty. Who is going to look after the child, and how will he follow up his wish for Docherty? This vignette illustrates the bond between the patient and the doctor, fused in an episode of care. It is similar to the scene in the first chapter of *Oliver Twist* by Charles Dickens where the mother dies after a difficult birth. As the doctor leaves he speaks to the nurse who has been drinking from a bottle.

'The old story' he said shaking his head, 'no wedding ring I see. Ah, good-night'. The medical gentlemen walked away to dinner. The nurse, having once more applied herself to the green bottle, sat down on a low chair by the fire, and proceeded to dress the infant[17].

The power of the word and the ability of the writer and the story to change attitudes and behaviour, and to make the reader think, are illustrated by the few extracts above. This is an aspect to which we will return later in the book.

The commonplace book

On several occasions in this introduction, the role of the commonplace book has been noted. This short section develops it further. The commonplace book is a collection of notes, writings and quotes kept by an individual, which reflects their interests and tastes, and provides a source of inspiration and enjoyment. It could be called a scrapbook, but it is not a diary. Records of such commonplace books are easy to find and provide an insight into the thinking and life of an individual.[18]

Robert Burns, for example, wrote two commonplace books and in his first he introduces it as follows.[19]

Observations, hints, songs, scraps of poetry etc., by Robt. Burness; a man who had little art in making money, and still less in keeping it; but was however, a man of some sense, a great deal of honesty, and unbounded good will to every creature – rational or irrational. As he was little indebted to scholastic education, and bred at the plough-tail, his performance must be strongly tinctured with his unpolished, rustic way of life; but as I believe

12

they are really his own, it may be some entertainment to a curious observer of human nature to see how a ploughman thinks and feels under the pressure of Love, Ambition, Anxiety, Grief, with the like cares and passions, which however diversified by the modes and manners of life, operate pretty much alike, I believe, in all the species.

In the pages which follow there are comments, songs, poems and ideas he had over the two year period. He notes, for example in March 1784 that:[20]

There was a certain period of my life that my spirit was broke by repeated losses and disasters, which threatened and indeed affected the utter ruin of my fortune. My Body too, was attacked by that most dreadful distemper, a hypochondria, or confirmed melancholy; in this wretched state, the recollection of which makes me yet shudder, I hung my harp on the willow trees, except in some lucid intervals in one of which I composed the following,

O Thou great being! What Thou are
Surpassest me to know
Yet sure I am, that known to thee
Are all affairs below

This is a very personal comment and deeply felt. Others first written in this commonplace book, are 'The death and Dyin' words o' poor Malie – my ain pet ewe – an unco mournful tale', and a letter sent to John Lapraik April 1st, 1785 in which he says:[21]

Gi'e me a'e spark o' nature's fire
That's a' the learning I desire.
Then tho' I drudge thro' dub and mire
 At pleugh or cart
My muse tho' hamely in attire
 May touch the heart

My own interest in a commonplace book began in the early 1960s when I found, as a medical student, in a now long-gone second-hand book shop in Glasgow, three volumes of *Horae Subsecivae*[22] by Dr John Brown, which contained the story of 'Rab and His Friends', quoted earlier in this introduction. Although I did not know at that time what a 'commonplace book' was, it was the beginning of a personal anthology and through notebooks to laptops I have kept lists of poems, titles, fragments of books, jokes and quotations. Over the years I have actively searched for pieces and quotes which have meant something special to me or which have triggered a piece of poetry or narrative.

Burns' commonplace book was written on eleven folio sheets, folded once to form a volume approximately 12½ inches by 7¾ inches. The 22 resultant sheets, 44 pages, composing the volume were once 'broached with a coarse thread', but later were richly bound in morocco.[23] It is much easier now to carry your commonplace book with you and have a mechanism to continue to add to your own notes. I go nowhere without a notebook and pen, or electronic notebook.

The purpose of the Commonplace is firstly, a personal record of what matters to you. Secondly, it will contain written word from a variety of sources which have provided some inspiration and cause for reflection, something to return to and enjoy. The third purpose is to record one's own thoughts for possible poems, articles and books. Such a personal resource can trigger new thinking and experiences.

It might be said that this is the kind of thing that academics do, and from which they can research and identify new areas to be explored. For medical students and those in the clinical professions, it provides a locus for personal interests and reflection. However the concept, and the audience, for the commonplace book is much wider than that. It can, and should, include the wider public, and in terms of clinical issues, patients and their families. They can be used for discussions, book clubs and for the greater understanding of the issues involved.

The reader of this book might like to consider what he or she might put in such a book to note their own special writings and sources of reflection.

Inevitably a book of this nature will provoke questions. Its genesis was to gain an understanding of the relationship between the makars and mediciners, between the poet and the doctor. It thus poses some questions to assist in giving direction and allow conclusions to be drawn at its end. These questions have been formed after a review of the widely available creative literature and relate to the discussion on quality of life, the determinants of health, and the practice of medicine. Links will also be made with contemporary medical literature and with the ways in which medical practitioners have been educated over the centuries. It also invites the reader to add to the poems, stories and novels used in this book.

Some of the questions are;

1. Is it possible, using contemporary Scottish literature, to identify factors which illustrate and illuminate medical practice, descriptions of illness and the determinants of health? Attitudes to death, and to quality of life, will be an important sub-set of this question. Does it provide a reality check between medical science, clinical practice, and the literature?
2. Are the characteristics of the doctor, and the broader health service, as displayed in the literature, effectively described and how these have changed (or not) over the years?
3. Is it possible through the literature to re-evaluate the value base of medicine? Can it help us to understand well-being and quality of life?
4. How can we identify learning opportunities that might enhance the study of health and of clinical practice, for both individuals and groups? Would a commonplace book be of value to students, practitioners, patients and the public?
5. How can stories be used to change attitudes and behaviour related to health?

The book is divided into a series of historical sections, and in each one there will be a short review of the major historical changes in Scotland to provide the wider context. This will include a link to important international events which had an impact on Scotland and to the major medical advances in the period, together with a comment on the educational opportunities available in Scotland and abroad. Finally, there will be a short summary and some general conclusions will be drawn.

Notes

1   K.C. Calman, R.S. Downie, M. Duthie, B. Sweeney, 'Literature and Medicine: A Course', *Medical Education*, 22 (1988), 265–69 and K.C. Calman and R.S. Downie, 'Why Arts Courses for Medicine?', *Lancet*, (1996), 1499–50.

2   M. Flinn (ed.), J. Gillespie, N. Hill, A. Maxwell, R. Mitchison, and C. Smout, *Scottish Population History from the 17th century to the 1930s* (Cambridge: Cambridge University Press, 1977), p. 295.

3   Ibid.

4   K.C. Calman, *A Study of Storytelling, Humour and Learning in Medicine* (London: The Stationery Office, 2000) and K.C. Calman, *Medical Education: Past, Present and Future* (Edinburgh: Elsevier, 2007).

5   Murray Pittock, personal communication, 2011.

6   Preamble to the Constitution of the World Health Organisation, Official Records of World Health Organisation, 10 (1946).

7   H.P. Tait, *A Doctor and Two Policemen: The History of the Edinburgh Health Department* (Edinburgh: Mackenzie and Storie, 1974).

8   K.C. Calman, *The Potential for Health* (Oxford: Oxford University Press, 1998).

9   Calman, *Storytelling, Humour and Learning in Medicine*.

10   K.C. Calman, 'Quality of Life in Cancer Patients', *Journal of Medical Ethics*, 228 (1984), 585–87.

11   Andrew Nash, *Kailyard and Scottish Literature* (Amsterdam: Rodopi, 2001).

12   Robert Henryson, 'The Abbey Walk' in Tom Scott (ed.), *The Penguin Book of Scottish Verse*, (London: Penguin Books, 1970), p. 84, ll. 4–11

13   Robert Burns, 'Address to the unco guid, or the rigidly righteous', (ll. 33–40) in James Mackay (ed.), *The Complete Poetical Works of Robert Burns* (Darvel: Alloway Publishing, 1993), pp.74–6.

14   Dr. John Brown, 'Rab and His Friends', in *Horae Subsecivae* (London: Adam and Charles Black, 1817), pp. 365–87

15   Ibid., p. 375.

16   William McIlvanney, *Docherty* (London: Sceptre Press, 1987), p. 25.

17   Charles Dickens, *The Complete Works*, Centennial Edition (Oxford: Oxford University Press, [n.d.]), p. 4.

18   Ann Moss, *Printed Commonplace Books* (Oxford: Oxford University Press, 1996) and R.D. Katzev, *In the Country of Books: Commonplace Books and other readings* (Matador, Leicester, 2009).

19   *Robert Burns' Commonplace Book, 1783–85,* ed. R.L. Brown, (Wakefield, England: S R Publishers Ltd, 1969).

20 Ibid, p. 11.

21 Ibid, p. 34.

22 John Brown, *Horae Subsecivae*, in three volumes (Series), (London: Adam and Charles Black, 1900).

23 Ibid, p. ii.

CHAPTER 2

Life is short and the Art long

The profession of medicine

To begin at the beginning. The title of this chapter comes from Hippocrates, the father of medicine, penned some 2,500 years ago, and is as true today as it was when it was written.

> Life is short, and the Art long; the occasion fleeting, experience fallacious and judgement difficult. The physician must not only be prepared to do what is right himself, but also to make the patient, the attendants, and the externals co-operate.[1]

The points he makes include the fact that it takes time and experience to learn medicine, and that it involves judgement. There is an 'art' to medicine. It emphasises the need to consider doing the right thing, the ethical dimension, and to involve the patient, and others, in the decision making process. This aphorism also highlights the two aspects of being a doctor which have been developed and written about in various ways and contexts over the centuries; the need for knowledge and experience, and an understanding of feelings, emotions and ethical issues: the science and the art. This is a very modern view of medical practice and it is at the heart of this book.

The problem, then, is how to ensure that doctors learn the things they need, put them into practice, and ensure full involvement of the patient. One way of exploring this very contemporary issue is to use the inspiration of the written word in the form of poems, novels, plays and fictional stories to illuminate the current roles and responsibilities of the doctor and other health professionals.

Since the time of Hippocrates in the 4th century BC, and presumably before, the medical profession has continually changed and developed. The last one hundred years have seen the most dramatic changes as the knowledge base has grown so rapidly and the ability to positively influence health has developed because of a strong and increasing evidence base. During this time there have been numerous discussions and debates on the values of the profession and the relationship between the art and the science of medicine.[2] This debate is even more focussed now as the expertise, knowledge and skills available to change lives has grown, and indeed continues to do so. Thus there is a constant need to re-assert and re-evaluate the humanity of the doctor. This includes the ethical issues which arise in clinical practice and the relationship, a very privileged one, between the patient and the doctor.

The medical profession itself has radically changed in terms of the knowledge base which is available, and this has resulted in changes to the process of medical education. The composition of the medical profession has also shifted over the 700 year period. Women medical students are now in the majority in medical schools, a complete change from the beginning of the 18th century. The first women graduates in Scotland did not appear until the end of the 19th century, and remained a small proportion of the total until relatively recently.[3]

Thus a consideration of the literature of Scotland provides one vehicle through which to examine these changes in health, medical practice and the rapidly expanding knowledge base. It also provides a way of considering the changes in the role of the doctor in society and may identify lessons for the education of doctors.

The aim of medicine

There has been considerable recent discussion on the role of medicine, its value base and the characteristics of the profession. With this in mind, what is the aim of medicine?

It is suggested that:

The aim of medicine is to assist in the process of healing in its broadest sense and it can apply to both individuals and communities. This is the

19

primary function of the doctor. Doctors do this by improving quality of life, providing care, relieving suffering, promoting health, preventing illness and disease. This aim is grounded in the understanding of health and the mechanisms of illness and disease and from this to provide effective and appropriate treatment. Finally doctors must do this in full co-operation with the patient, public and other providers of health care.[4]

Put another way, the purpose of medicine is to serve the community by continually improving health, health care, and quality of life, for the individual and the population, by understanding disease, promoting health, prevention of illness, treatment and care, and the effective use of resources, all within the context of a team approach.

There is a philosophical issue around such aims. Are they timeless, or do they change as the environment, culture and knowledge base changes? Presented as in the statements above the general aims could be seen to be long lasting and then interpreted and modified in the more detailed objectives of the doctor at any particular time.

The roles of the doctor

Several roles thus follow from the aim set out above:

- To be a healer, understand the processes of care and to intervene when appropriate. To wish to help others and see medicine as a vocation. To work as part of a team.
- To understand people, and use this to provide better care, with co-operation and involvement of the patient and the public, should they wish. To communicate as effectively as possible. To be an advocate for health.
- To understand the reasons for illness and disease and to use this knowledge to improve health, health care and improved quality of life and well-being. Medicine is an art as well as a science.

The kind of doctor required is one whose qualities fit these roles; that of healer, people centred, and curious about health and illness. By defining the qualities required, not the type of doctor, it becomes easier to define what a doctor should be.

These then are some of the characteristics of a profession, though there are some who would argue that in the 21st century medicine is no more than a trade, a series of skills which can be easily mastered and bought at a price. This is not what a profession should be. It has at its core a commitment to people and has a strong vocational aspect without which it would just be another job. It follows from this that respect for the value of human life is a given, as is privacy and confidentiality. Acting as an advocate may seem again to be out of place, but, as will be discussed in another section, it is increasingly important. Perhaps the most contentious is that the profession should sets its own standards and be self-regulating. In the 21st century the public should be part of this and self-regulation could be seen to perpetuate an inward-looking club, with no responsibility to the public. But these views are not incompatible. The public involvement in such bodies as the General Medical Council and increasingly in the Medical Royal Colleges provides a way in which such an input can occur. The profession of medicine should not be afraid of such ventures as they can only strengthen the profession when those outside see the effort involved. As Freidson noted, Medicine should not be without lay evaluation.[5]

Some writings on the science and value base of medicine

The two cornerstones of medical practice, science and ethics, are at the heart of the professional role of the doctor, and both relate to clinical practice and to improving public health. This short section describes a few of the writings on this topic that are of particular relevance to the wider debate and which have had some influence in the generation and formulation of this book.

This section also defines some of the criteria by which the extracts from the literature of Scotland, noted in this book, can be judged. These criteria include the dual function of the doctor as a scientist and a humane person, the importance of quality of life, the importance of health promotion, the need for certain characteristics in the 'good doctor' and the importance of learning and thinking.

21

It is interesting to note that doctors from all generations have had an interest in the arts, and have been successful novelists and poets, and this broad theme is one which has been told many times. Scottish doctors who have achieved a reputation in writing include: Arthur Johnston (1587–1641), Patrick Abercromby (1656–1716), John Arbuthnott (1667–1735), David Moir (1798–1857), Tobias Smollett (1721–1771), Arthur Conan Doyle (1859–1930), James Bridie (O.H.Mavor) (1888–1951), A.J.Cronin (1896–1981), Ronald David Laing (1927–1989), Colin Douglas (1945–), Anne MacLeod (1951–), Alexander McCall Smith (1948–) and Iain Bamforth (1959–). Some, but not all, may use their clinical background in their non-medical writing, and there is, of course, an ethical question here in relation to confidentiality. All writers, probably, use their life experience of course, and, no doubt, some of those just listed do so.

It is of interest that Robert Louis Stevenson considered the role of the doctor in his dedication to *Underwoods and Ballads* (1894) and this will be discussed in more detail later in the book. He notes:

> There are men and classes of men that stand above the common herd: the soldier, the sailor, and the shepherd not infrequently; the artist rarely; rarer still, the clergyman; and the physician almost as a rule. He is the flower (such as it is) of our civilisation; and when that stage of man is done with, and only to be marvelled at in history, he will be thought to have shared as little, as any in the defects of the period, and most notably exhibited the virtues of the race. Generosity he has, such as is possible to those who practice an art, never to those who drive a trade; discretion, tested by a hundred secrets; tact, tried in a thousand embarrassments; and what are more important, Herculean cheerfulness and courage. So that he brings air and cheer into the sick room, and often enough, though not as often as he wishes, brings healing[6]

Earlier Francis Bacon sets out a similar wide remit for the medical person and all those interested in learning. In *The Advancement of Learning* Bacon details the two books which are required for study if we are 'to be secured from error'.[7] He states that these books are 'first the scriptures and then the creatures expressing his power', the books of ethics and of nature. In his book *Novum Organum* he comments in particular on the problems in the advancement of the sciences: 'By far the greatest obstacle to the advancement of the sciences, and the undertaking of any new attempt or department, is to be found in men's despair and the idea of impossibility.'[8] He concludes that new thinking is possible, but requires hope and imagination. He develops the knowledge theme further as he suggests:

> Man, as the minister and interpreter of nature, does and understands as much as his observations on the order of nature, either with regard to things or the mind, permit him, and neither knows nor is capable of more.[9]

So how can man learn more? 'The human understanding is most excited by that which strikes and enters the mind at once and suddenly, and by which the imagination is immediately filled and inflated.'[10]

Thus new knowledge is important and 'knowledge and human power are synonymous, since ignorance of the cause frustrates the effect.'[11] The power of contemporary medical knowledge has been enhanced greatly over the years, and in dealing with the sick and distressed the power of the physician also enhanced; hence the need for the second aspect of the medical role, that of considering the hopes and feelings and wishes of the patient.

Janis McLaren Caldwell, in her book *Literature and medicine in nineteenth century Britain: From Mary Shelly to George Eliot,*[12] picks up this same theme and she describes the rapid changes in medical practice in the 19th century moving away from the basic task of taking a history from the patient, to the introduction of a formal clinical examination which is ultimately based on an understanding of pathology. These two aspects on which clinical practice was based at the time, history taking and clinical examination, she calls 'romantic realism'. She draws attention to what we might think of as contrasting ideas, evidence and imagination, and highlights, in fact, the contribution of these two sides of 19th century literature and demonstrates that it is the combination of the two sides of clinical practice, the science and the personal, which is central to the role of the doctor as seen in the literature.

Oliver Wendell Holmes (1809–1894)

Holmes was a physician in Boston at the end of the 19th century and taught at Dartmouth Medical College and Harvard, where he was Dean, and wrote a series of books and lectures on a variety of medical subjects. His most widely read were a series of notes entitled *The Professor at the Breakfast Table* (1859), *The Autocrat at the Breakfast Table* (1858) and others. They all show considerable erudition, wide reading and a concept of the doctor as a humane person, as well as a scientist. One of his major insights was into quality of life. This quotation from *The Professor at the Breakfast Table* summarises well the problem of thinking about people in a simplistic way:

> The longer I live the more I am satisfied of two things; first, that the truest lives are those that are cut rose diamond fashion, with many facets, answering to the many-planed aspects of the world about them; secondly, that society is always trying in some way or another to grind us down to a single flat surface.[13]

Such a statement serves to emphasise the need to consider the whole person in the clinical encounter, and not just think of the patient as a series of symptoms and signs which need a solution.

Sir William Osler (1849–1919)

Sir William Osler was perhaps the doyen of medical writers and brought together a remarkable range of thinking and writing. He was foundation Professor of Medicine at Johns Hopkins Medical School in Baltimore (1889–1905), and Regius Professor of Medicine in Oxford (1905–1919). He wrote a classic textbook of medicine, *The Principles and Practice of Medicine*.[14] In the 1921 edition there is a preface by Thomas McCrae, who makes the point that the 'Textbook' was one of the great interests in Osler's life. Osler had said that it brought him 'Mind to Mind' with members of the profession in many parts of the world, passing on not only medical knowledge but attitudes and a way of life.[15] To Osler the textbook was more than just a source of data and information, but an opportunity to express a philosophy and attitude as a doctor.

His great writings include *Aequanimitas*, *The Collection of a Library*, *Books and Men*, *The Master-Word in Medicine* and *Teaching and Thinking*. More than any other individual he brought together the two aspects of medicine, raised earlier, those of science and the humanities as essays or as speeches to students and staff. The following are some pertinent extracts from his writings.

From *Aequanimitas:*[16]

> An old writer says that there are four sorts of readers: 'sponges which attract all without distinguishing; Howre-glasses receive and pour out as fast; bagges which only retain the dregges of the spices and let the wine escape, and Sives which retain the best onely.' A man wastes a great many years before he reaches the 'sive' stage.

It is hard for me to speak of the value of libraries in terms which would not seem exaggerated. Books have been my delight these thirty years, and from them I have received incalculable benefits. To study the phenomenon of disease without books is to sail an uncharted sea, while to study books without patients is not to go to sea at all . . . For the teacher a great library is indispensable. They must know the best work and know it at once. They mint and make current coin the ore so widely scattered in journals, transactions and monographs.

From *The Student Life:*[17]

> The all-important thing is to get a relish for the good company of the race in a daily intercourse with some of the great minds of all ages. Now in the spring-time of life, pick your inmates from among them, and begin a systematic cultivation of their works . . . Start at once a bed side library and spend the last half hour of the day in the communion with the saints of humanity . . . A library represents the mind of its collector, his fancies, foibles, his strengths and weaknesses, his prejudices and preferences.

The humanities are the hormones. I like to think of the pleasant-flavoured word as embracing all the knowledge of the ancient classical world – what man knew of Nature as well as what he knew of himself.

The critical sense and sceptical attitude of the Hippocratic School laid the foundations of modern medicine on broad lines, and we owe to it: first, the emancipation of medicine from the shackles of priest-craft and of caste; secondly, the conception of medicine as an art based on accurate observation, and as a science, an integral part of the science of man and nature; Thirdly, the high moral ideal, expressed in that most memorable of documents, the Hippocratic Oath; the conception and realisation of medicine as the profession of a cultivated gentleman.

To carefully observe the phenomenon of life in all its phases, normal and perverted, to make perfect that most difficult of all arts, the art of observation, to call to the aid the science of experimentation, to cultivate the reasoning faculty, so to be able to know the true from the false – these are our methods. To prevent disease, to relieve suffering and to heal the sick-this is our work.

This quotation raises the issue of professionalism in medicine and is one which will be discussed in more detail later.

Finally, William Osler lists his personal ideals:

I have had three personal ideals. One, to do the day's work well and not bother about tomorrow. . . . The second ideal has been to act the Golden Rule, as far as in me lay, towards my professional brethren and towards the patients committed to my care. And the third has been to cultivate such a measure of equanimity as would enable me to bear success with humility, the affection of my friends with pride and to be ready when the day of sorrow and grief come to meet it with the courage befitting of a man.

These were the final words of William Osler when he addressed the Profession of United States and Canada at the farewell dinner in New York, May 2nd

1904. It will be interesting to see how these words are, or are not, reflected in the role of the doctor in Scottish literature.

Sir William Tennant Gairdner (1824–1902)

Sir William Tennant Gairdner was both Professor of Medicine in Glasgow and the first Medical Officer of Health in that city. He wrote in a similar vein to Osler, but he had an added public health dimension. It is interesting to note that it was he who introduced 'ticketing' in Glasgow slums, a subject which will be raised later, as it involved placing a 'ticket' outside a home, or a room indicating how many people should live in the space. He was also concerned that doctors, as they specialise, will lose interest in the wider determinants of health:

> The limitation of sanitary functions to men not engaged in medical practice, and of the practice of medicine and surgery to persons who are, or may conceive themselves to be, thereby exempt from all preventative duty, will not be without serious disadvantages. It will tend to split up the medical profession into sections, perhaps into two more or less hostile camps . . . For the healing art is really, in a very practical sense, one; and the cure of disease, if it is to be anything else than mere empiricism, must be largely imbued with a preventative element. In other words, the careful and practical study of the causes of disease with a view to prevention is in many, if not in most, cases a large part of the cure.[18]

With Gairdner we find an expression of the wider role of the doctor, not to deal only with individual people (patients), but also of their responsibility to the wider community and the health of the public.

Paul Tournier (1898–1986)

Tournier was both a physician and an ethicist with wide experience of caring for people. In his remarkable book *Creative Suffering* (1983) Tournier develops the concept that we have all suffered and had problems and that the real issue is what we do with the suffering. He says, 'Events give us joy or pain, but our growth is determined by our personal response to both, by our inner attitude.' He goes further 'there is a double task for the doctor; to work towards healing, and to help the patient make, in Pascal's words, good use of his sickness.'[19] In this short sentence he crystallises two of the key features of medicine, providing ways of helping the patient to get better, and that of assisting the patient to benefit from his or her illness. Thus the warp and the woof of clinical practice – the science and the art, are both relevant and should be focussed on healing the patient, and of communicating with the patient and relatives. In public health terms this relates both to the hard science and to the equally difficult, and in some ways more difficult, sphere of public opinion. The balance of these two cultures changes with the knowledge base and this leads us to understand the necessity of a wider and richer context for the discussion of the profession of medicine, ranging widely beyond that of merely 'empirical' or 'scientific' concerns.

G. Gregory Smith

Finally, as a quite different example of the two aspects of life as expressed in literature, the writings of G. Gregory Smith are relevant. In his book *Scottish Literature: Character and influence* (1919) he introduced the term 'Caledonian Antisyzigy' to illustrate two dimensions in Scottish literature that he considered to be important.[20] The first he characterises as realism, a sense of detail, a grasp of the facts. This is about close observation, and 'by a cummulation of touches a quick and perfect image is presented to the reader.' The second is the role of the senses 'in the fun of things thrown topsy-turvy in the norms of Elfland and the voices of the mountains'.[21] In essence it is the contrast between real life and romance. He calls these two aspects the warp and the woof of literature and provides for us a remarkably interesting way of describing clinical practice, whose warp and woof are science and the arts. Although not consciously concerned with medicine in literature, Gregory Smith's identified dualism is a nice 'diagnosis' of how literature, indeed humanity, operates as fully in the imaginative as in the empirical realm and this dualism exists naturally in fully functioning clinical practice. It

28

highlights a 'medical antisyzigy' in which the dual attributes of the doctor, knowledge and the humanity, are woven together; the warp and the woof of clinical practice.

It is with this wider theme of the rich context in which medical practice should be viewed, that this book is concerned.

Notes

1   Hippocrates, 'Aphorism 1', in *The Genuine Works of Hippocrates*, trans. Francis Adams (Baltimore: William and Wilkins, 1939), p. 292.

2   K.C. Calman, 'The Profession of Medicine', *British Medical Journal*, (1994), 1140–3.

3   Kate Campbell Hurd-Mead, *A History of Women in Medicine* (New York: AMS Press, 1977); Ruth Fox Hume, *Great Women in Medicine* (New York: Random House, 1964); Elizabeth Blackwell, *Pioneering Work in Opening the Medical Profession to Women* (London: Longmans Green and Co, 1895); Ted Grant and Sandy Carter, *Women in Medicine: A Celebration of Their Work* (Ontario: Firefly Books, 2004).

4   Calman, *Medical Education*, p. 347.

5   E. Friedson, 'The Limits of Professional Autonomy', in *Profession of Medicine* (New York: Dodd, Mead and Company, 1975), pp. 335–58.

6   Robert Louis Stevenson, 'Dedication', *Underwoods and Ballads* (Charleston: Bibliobazaar, 2006), p. 13.

7   Francis Bacon, *The Advancement of Learning, Novum Organum, New Atlantis* (Chicago: William Benton, 1952), I, p. 125.

8   Ibid, p. 125.

9   Ibid, p. 107.

10 Ibid, p. 110.

11 Ibid, p. 107.

12 Janis McLaren Caldwell, *Literature and Medicine in Nineteenth Century Britain: From Mary Shelley to George Eliot* (Cambridge: Cambridge University Press, 2004).

13 Oliver Wendell Holmes, *The Professor at the Breakfast Table* (London: Routledge, 1905), p. 29.

14 Sir William Osler, *The Principles and Practice of Medicine*, 9th edn (New York: B. Appleton and Co., 1921).

15 Ibid, p. vii.

16 William Osler, *Aequanimitas, With Other Addresses* (London: H.K. Lewis, 1904).

17 Sir William Osler, *The Student Life: The Philosophy of William Osler*, ed. R.E. Verney (Edinburgh: E and S Livingstone, 1957).

18 Sir William Tennant Gairdner, *The Physician as Naturalist* (Glasgow: James Maclehose, 1889), p. 277.

19 Paul Tournier, *Creative Suffering* (San Francisco: Harper Row Publishing, 1983), p. 29.

20 G. Gregory Smith, *Scottish Literature: Character and Influence* (London: MacMillan and Co., 1919), p. 4.

21 Ibid, p. 19.

CHAPTER 3

A short history of Scotland

The history of Scotland from the 14th century to the present

We are generally at a loss to conceive how mankind can subsist under manners and customs extremely different from our own; and we are apt to exaggerate the misery of barbarous times, by an imagination of what we ourselves should suffer in a situation to which we are not accustomed. But every age hath its consolations, as well as its sufferings.

Adam Ferguson (1767)[1]

Much has been written on the history of Scotland during the last 700 years. In the context of this book the stories behind the history set the scene for the understanding of the place, time and medical background to the work under consideration. This short section will emphasise, in particular, those aspects of Scottish history which might affect the determinants of health, and the practice of medicine. The history of medicine in Scotland is well covered in other writings.[2]

Change and the 'Common Man'

Between the 14th and 17th centuries three major changes occurred which have had significant long-term implications. First the Wars of Independence, with the national heroes of Wallace and Bruce, the Declaration of Arbroath in 1320 and the subsequent continuing conflict between the two nations. Then there was the Reformation in the middle of the 16th century which changed the character of the people of Scotland and had a significant impact on education. The Union of the Crowns in 1603 was followed by the deposition of Charles I by Cromwell and then the Restoration in 1660 and finally the Union of the Parliaments in 1707. In the early centuries it was a violent

31

time, and dominated by the Three Estates; the hierarchy of the church, the nobility and the Burgh representatives. The 'Common Man' had no real place in the organisation of the State. Illness was common with infections such as smallpox and the plague being particularly rife. Mortality was high, and childhood deaths and death in pregnancy a major problem. Famine was also a regular feature across the population

Medical care was limited and remedies few and generally ineffective. However during this period Scotland inaugurated five universities; St Andrews (1411), Glasgow (1451), Aberdeen (1495), Edinburgh (1583) and Marischal College (1593) and three medical colleges, the Royal College of Surgeons of Edinburgh (1505), Royal College of Physicians and Surgeons of Glasgow (1599), and the Royal College of Physicians of Edinburgh in 1681, and they began to award medical degrees. Scotland also had a medical kindred in the family of the Beatons, the physicians to the Lords of the Isles and to the Kings of Scotland. This story will be expanded later.

As the 18th century dawned the significance of the constitutional changes became clear. Scotland began in 1700 as a country within a United Kingdom, but with its own Parliament, and seven years later in 1707, the parliaments were united. Over a long period the case for a Scottish Parliament grew. In 1997 a referendum was called, which re-instated the Scottish Parliament in 1999, and the story continues. Such a series of changes, embedded in the literature of Scotland and the 'auld sang' is still on-going.

Conflict has never been far from the surface. The Jacobite rebellions in 1715 and 1745 left a lasting legacy in song, verse and story. Scots were involved in the Napoleonic wars, the Crimean War, the Boer War, two major conflicts in the 20th century, in current conflicts, and much in between. The Scottish soldier as a folk hero, and the reflection on battles and their causes remains an important aspect of Scottish writing with roots that pre-date the 18th century, but which become particularly prominent from that time.

It is perhaps social and economic change which has seen the greatest movement. In the beginning of the 18th century Scotland was largely a rural economy. People worked on the land and lived where they were born. Education was limited and there was an expectation that the social class you were born in would be where you stayed. This is well reflected in Thomas Johnston's *History of the Working Classes in Scotland* (1929).[3] The key individuals in the local community were the laird, the minister, the school teacher or dominie, and the local doctor.

With the coming of the Industrial Revolution in the 19th century, much of it generated in Scotland, everything changed and the population moved and grew, old values were lost, housing and social conditions in many cases worsened, and there was a rise in a new middle class. Cities like Glasgow developed hugely: it changed its character from a small cathedral and uni-versity town to the second city of the Empire. Paisley, Greenock and towns in Lanarkshire did the same. In Edinburgh the growth of the New Town changed again the character of the city and in Dundee the new industries, such as jute, meant expansion and growth. By the beginning of the 20th century the life of people had changed out of all recognition.

Reform, education and socio-economic factors

Social reformers tried to change the pattern of growth and quality of life, and new models of living were introduced in response to some of the negative aspects of change. One the of most interesting was in New Lanark where Robert Owen and David Dale created an entirely new way of living providing work, education and religion in the one place. The novel *Margaret Maitland* by Margaret Oliphant reflects this development, and will be dis-cussed later.

The education system also changed with parish schools still able to cope in the rural areas, but significant changes were required in towns. 'The Ragged Schools', championed by Thomas Guthrie were established and these looked after poor children, often orphans, and were replicated elsewhere to deal with child education; William Quarrier introduced his orphanages to deal with another aspect of the problem. The working conditions of children and adults in many of the new industries were awful, and it took time and the passionate concerns of many to change these. Associated with these changes were major health and safety issues, whether in factories or in the expanding coal mining sector. Edwin Muir vividly described the atmosphere in *The Story and the Fable* when he was a clerk in a Greenock bone factory at the beginning of the 20th century:

Sometimes he fancied that the smell always clung to him, that it had soaked into his skin and went about with him like a corrupt aura. He had heard that the men and women, who worked in the yard, unloading the bones and casting them into the furnace, never got rid of the smell, no matter how they scrubbed. It got among the women's hair and into the pores of their skin. It breathed into the faces of their lovers when at night, under the hawthorn bushes outside the town, they found a few moments of sensual forgetfulness, they breathed it out with their last breath, infecting the host which the priest set between their lips, and making it taste of McClintock's bone factory. A thing so tenacious and vile had given him at first a feeling of mystical revulsion, but he had got used to it.[4]

In factories, especially those that dealt with chemicals, poisoning with lead and mercury often occurred but were slowly subject to legislation and the incidence of such problems declined.

Within the literature of Scotland these changes are reflected and commented on and show the impact on health and welfare, and, as social and economic factors are a major driver and determinant of health, they became a major factor in the poor health which Scotland enjoyed. Slum conditions were very bad and overcrowding and poverty became breeding grounds for disease. A glance through the volume *A study of the diet of the labouring classes in Edinburgh* [5] shows just how shocking the conditions were. The practice of 'ticketing' (that was mentioned earlier) was adopted and determined how many people might sleep in a room; these tickets were placed at the door and the room was subject to regular inspection. As the slums developed so the middle classes moved out to suburbs and villas, away from the grime and smoke. The rise in the middle classes was also associated with philanthropy and schools, universities, art galleries and museums, hospitals and many other institutions were established in this way. In the words of Andrew Carnegie (1835–1919), a multi-millionaire philanthropist born in Dunfermline, but who made his fortune in steel in the United States of America, it was the 'Gospel of Wealth', to give away the wealth you had made for the benefit of others.[6]

In the middle of this change, Scotland was the home of the Enlightenment, predominantly in Edinburgh. Here the intellectual achievements of Hume, Smith, Ferguson, Kames, Stewart and many others gained a worldwide reputation. The Faculty of Medicine in Edinburgh in the late 18th century, grown out of the great school in Leyden, became the greatest medical school of the age, and began a medical tradition in Scotland which has lasted until the present. Newspapers and journals developed and circulating libraries brought news and new ideas. As literacy developed so these ideas became more important and during some of the unrest in the 19th century the literate and well educated weavers were at the heart of the protests.

Behaviour and lifestyle

Other factors which determine health are personal behaviour and lifestyle. As the 18th-century opened, most, other than the upper classes, ate potatoes, oats and fish. Very little meat was consumed and the diet was plain and simple. They walked everywhere and there was little public transport. Alcohol was a problem, with many stories of overindulgence, and the illegitimacy rates were high. There was no issue with cigarette smoking or the use of hard drugs, and obesity was confined to a small group of the population, generally the rich. Contrast this with the end of the 20th century with high cigarette smoking rates, obesity and drug-related issues and, for many, lack of regular exercise. In between there were many issues all well recorded in the novels and poetry of the Nation, and in the public movements and laws which sought to change these conditions. For alcohol, the Band of Hope and the Children's Temperance Movement, the Forbes MacKenzie Act of 1853, which banned drinking in licensed premises on Sunday's, and increasing the taxes on alcohol, beginning in 1909, made a significant difference. The rise of the Prohibitionist Party, whose candidate Edwin Scrymgeour beat Winston Churchill in Dundee in 1924, all added to the remarkable changes which were occurring and which show how important individuals were in changing the habits of the nation.

The biggest single change in improving health and welfare occurred after the Second World War in 1945 with the creation of the welfare state and the National Health Service.

Throughout the 700 year period the role and status of religion also changed significantly. At the beginning of the period Scotland was a country whose religion was Roman Catholicism and following the Protestant Reformation in the 16th century it became strictly Calvanist, with the Book of Discipline central to the ethos of the population. The local minister was important and powerful, as is amply demonstrated in the literature of Scotland and which will be discussed later. Sunday schools provided both an education and a grounding in the faith. The Disruption of 1843 was a major event which tore the church in two, and reflected the real feelings of the minister and members. But as the population moved into cities, and grew, there was a need for something different; missions and new ways of delivering the message developed. Reforming ministers such as Thomas Chalmers in the 19th century, and more recently Tom Allan and Geoff Shaw in the 20th century, were a major force for change. In Glasgow for example the Boys' Brigade, founded in 1883, began as a way of helping boys in the community to find something to do rather than fight in the streets, backed by a Christian message. As time passed the relevance of the Church and the influx, mainly in the west of Scotland, of Irish Catholics, raised the spectrum of sectarianism which, along with violence, has remained a problem to the present day; both of which are reflected in the literature. For sport, football remains a major passion, both playing and watching, and golf as a local Scottish sport still has great popularity. The first Scottish football team was Queens Park in 1867 with Ayr and Partick Thistle following in 1868.

The political map also changed with implications beyond Scotland. In figures such as Keir Hardie, James Maxton and the Red Clydesiders the political ethos moved sharply to the left and the foundation of the Scottish Labour Party and the Independent Labour Party changed not only Scotland, but the Westminster Parliament.

The practice of medicine

Medical developments over the 700 year period have been huge, and have changed the role and ability of the doctor as a healer. First there have been major changes in the education and regulation of doctors. At the beginning of the period under consideration, qualification was a loose matter, many not bothering to take the university degree, or in the earliest period, any degree at all. The Medical Royal Colleges and Faculties provided an alternative route to practice. It was the concern of patients and the public about the qualifications and competence of the doctor that brought about the establishment of the General Medical Council in 1858. Subsequently this basic registration has been expanded and now includes specialty practice.

The second major change has been in the organisation of medical practice. With little in the therapeutic armamentarium, most doctors were generalists, with a few having special interests in such things as surgery and obstetrics. However with the new medical knowledge driving the changes, specialisation (including in general practice) has become the norm. This is readily reflected in the literature of Scotland particularly in the 20th century.

The major driver for change has been in the creation of new scientific knowledge, and Scotland has played a significant role in such developments. In the middle of the 18th century there were few effective drugs and diagnostic techniques were very limited. Developments in Paris in particular opened up a new way of investigating patients using a stethoscope, percussion and palpation. These became even more relevant with developments in pathology and bacteriology, which allowed the clinical findings to be related to what might actually be happening in the body. Disease categorisation changed, and there was much more for the student to learn. Dissection was not just about anatomy but about what caused disease in the first place, add to these developments in antisepsis and anaesthesia, and all changed; surgical techniques expanded, and new procedures were created; research became possible, and the evidence base for new and old treatments came under scrutiny. Antibiotics and others drugs followed, and diseases which had been untreatable were able to be cured. By 1953 the genetic code had been cracked and the therapeutic benefits continue to be seen. New methods of visualising the body were discovered, beginning with X-rays and moving to ultrasound, computerised tomography (CT) and magnestic resonance imaging (MRI) scans. Even in my clinical lifetime, the change has been substantial and is increasing daily.

Public health medicine became a major force for change and public health measures included clean water (as in the introduction of the Water Works Act in Glasgow in 1855 when for the first time in Britain clean water was brought from Loch Katrine to Glasgow at huge cost), clean air (as in the Clean Air Act of 1956 following the great smog of 1952), immunisation programmes and efforts to change behaviour, such as cigarette smoking and diet. Life span has increased enormously over the period, readily seen in the figures in childhood mortality.

On more than one occasion it has been emphasised that this increase in knowledge and the expanding evidence base has significantly changed the role of the doctor and with it the relationship between the doctor and the patient. Rather than decreasing the non-science side of medicine, it has increased it in proportion. Ethical issues, for example are now much more openly discussed, and competence and medical behaviour readily questioned. Courses on ethics and communication skills are the norm nowadays, and clinical skills laboratories help equip the young doctor to deal with the problems they will face.

Notes

1   Adam Ferguson, *Essay on the History of Civil Society*, ed. Fania Oz-Salzberger (London: Transaction Publications, 1995), pp. 103–4.

2   J.D. Comrie *History of Scottish Medicine* in Two Volumes (London: Bailliere, Tindall and Cox, 1932); D. Hamilton. *The Healers: A History of Medicine in Scotland* (Edinburgh: Cannongate, 1981); H. Dingwall, D. Hamilton, I. Macintyre, M. McCrae, D. Wright, *Scottish Medicine: An Illustrated History* (Edinburgh: Birlinn, 2011).

3   Thomas Johnston, *History of the Working Classes in Scotland* (Glasgow: Forward, 1929).

4   Edwin Muir, *The Story and the Fable* (London: G.G. Harran and Co., 1940), pp. 163–4.

5   D.N. Paton, J.C. Dunlop, E. Inglis, *A Study of the Diet of the Laboring Classes in Edinburgh* (Edinburgh: Otto Schulte and Company, 1906).

6   Andrew Carnegie, *The Gospel of Wealth and Other Timely Essays*, 3rd edn (London: Frederick Warne, 1903), p. 24.

Chapter 4

The early history of Scotland;

Kingdoms, religion, makars and mediciners.

The period of four centuries between the battle of Bannockburn in June 1314 and the Union of the Parliaments in 1707 was a turbulent and violent time, beginning with the Wars of Independence, in which the two great heroes, William Wallace and Robert the Bruce, dominated the scene. Both were celebrated in verse, and Blind Harry's long poem 'Wallace'[1] demonstrates just how violent it was: battles, ambushes, killings, burnings and violent deaths. The country was dominated by the 'Three Estates', the nobility, the church and the merchant class and there was no role for the common people. The enmity with England remained and indeed was strengthened by the Declaration of Arbroath in 1320, and the links with France grew through trade and royal marriage.

Many of the events are recorded in the literature, which was predominantly poetry and ballads, with some plays, but little prose writing; it was the age of the makars with names such as Henryson, Dunbar and William Drummond.

By the middle of the 16th century the second major change occurred, that of the Protestant Reformation of the church, following the pattern in Europe, though different and distinct from the Reformation in England. The consequences had a profound effect on the people of Scotland, in several different ways. Firstly, there was the call to establish a church in each parish and a General Assembly which gave the people of Scotland a place to meet and debate. It provided an alternative parliament. Secondly, the Book of Discipline provided an impetus for education in schools and universities, which, though it took time to evolve, resulted in significant change and improvement. For example in the Book of Discipline written in 1560 by John Knox it states;

Of necessitie therefore we judge it, that every severall Kirk have one school-maister appointed, such a one at least as is able to teach Grammer and the Latine tongue if the town be of any reputation. If it be upaland [rural] . . .then must either a reader or the minister there be appointed to take care over the children and youth of the parish, to instruct them in the first rudiments and especially in the Catechisme. . ...And furder we think it expedient that in in any notable town there be erected a Colledge, in which the arts, at least Logick and Rhetorick, and the tongues, be read by sufficient masters, for whom honest stipends must be appointed. . ...Last the great Schooles, called the universities, shall be replenished with these that shall bee apt to learning.

Such Universities did flourish, as will be discussed shortly. The third document of significance was the Confession of Faith,[2] again composed in 1560 by Knox and the church. In it there is a statement of 'Quhat Warkis ar Reputed Gude befoir God'. They are of two sorts; the first is to honour God and the second for the good of our neighbours. This meant to honour your father and mother, princes and superior powers, to save the lives of innocents, to defend the oppressed, to keep our bodies clean and healthy, to live in soberness and temperance, and to deal justly with all men, in both word and deed, and finally to repress all appetite to hurt our neighbours.

The health of the population at this time was poor and dominated by infection and periods of famine. Plague, smallpox and leprosy figure highly, and Robert the Bruce is said to have had leprosy. It is interesting to note therefore, that around this period, just before the Reformation another document appeared, 'The Complaynt of Scotland' an 'Epistil to the Quenis Grace', an exhortation to the Three Estates to be vigilant in defence of their public role. It was written to Queen Mary of Guise and contains the following words in the first page of the document.[3]

The special cause of our affliction has precedit of the three vehement plagis quilk has al maist succumbit oure cuntre in final euertione, that is to saye, the cruel invasions of oure ald enemesi, the universal pestilence, ande mortalite, that has occurit mercyles amang the people and the contentions diverse of the thre estatis of Scotland.

40

The document acknowledged that pestilence had been as great a problem as the English invasions and the divisions amongst the Three Estates. The population of Scotland at this time was small, perhaps less than 800,000, and any loss of life would have been very significant. Infant deaths and deaths in childbirth were also common.

It was also the beginning of smoking tobacco and King James VI, only son of Mary Queen of Scots, who acceded to the throne of England in 1603, uniting the Crowns of the two countries, wrote on the topic. He was one of the first to comment on the effect of smoking on health and a year after the accession, in 1604, he wrote an essay entitled 'A Counterblaste to Tobacco'. In it he sets out why people might want to smoke, for example, it might help to cure diease. He says:

> Tobacco being a common herbe was first found to be a preservative, or antidot against the Pockes . . . It cures gowt in the feet . . . it makes a man sober that was drunke . . . it makes one sleepe soundly, yet being taken when a man is drowsie, it will as they say, awake his braine . . . Oh omnipotent power of Tobacco!

He notes that offering tobacco is the common way of greeting a friend. He ends with an unforgettable statement:

> A custome loathsome to the eye, hatefull to the Nose, harmefull to the braine, dangerous to the Lungs, and the black stinking fume thereof, neerest resembling the horrible Stigian smoke of the pit that is bottomelesse.

The third major event relates to the constitutional issues including the deposition of Charles I, the Commonwealth of Cromwell and the restoration of the monarchy, coupled with the Union of the Crowns in 1603 and the Union of the Parliaments in 1707. Once again these changes had a significant influence on the character of Scotland at the time and into succeeding centuries.

Associated with this period were the Covenanters, a group of Scots who, over the 16th and 17th centuries, signed a series of Covenants to prevent the interference of the Stuart Kings in the affairs of the Church of Scotland

and the imposition of the Book of Common Prayer. The National Covenant was signed in 1638 in the Kirkyard of Greyfriars Church in Edinburgh. The movement was associated with a range of battles and methods of resistance such as the Conventicles with outdoor preaching. The Cameronians, named after the Reverend Richard Cameron, was a more extreme group. The movement came to an end, but not completely, in the reign of William of Orange and had links into the Jacobite Rising.

In terms of clinical practice little changed. Practitioners were rarely qualified and though as the centuries passed the university influence grew there was no real need to be formally qualified. Aberdeen University for example had the first chair in Medicine in the English speaking world (1497), and from the early 18th century onwards degrees were awarded by both Glasgow and Edinburgh Universities. The Medical Royal Colleges were also important as sources of education and experience.

Of particular interest in the Western Isles of Scotland were a group of medical practitioners who formed a 'medical kindred profession' and who were the hereditary physicians to the Lords of the Isles, the Beatons.[4] The name is spelled differently at different times but include Macbeth, and Bethune. The earliest on record is Patrick Macbeth, *capitilis medicus surgerie* to Robert I, King of Scots. The medical interest in this family is in their education, which is directly linked to the great Medical School in Salerno, the greatest medical school in Europe in the 13th century. Manuscripts survive which make the direct link, and include the works of Avicenna, Bernardus Gordon and Hippocrates. These were translated into Gaelic and thus Gaelic joins Greek, Latin and Arabic as one of only four languages in which this great body of knowledge was formally and systematically studied and taught. The work of the Beatons is described in a book by Martin Martin, *A Description of the Western Isles of Scotland* written in 1695. In it he describes meeting some of the Beatons and describes some of the treatments used.[5] He comments on leprosy, ague/malaria, smallpox and the use, for example, of sea plants as treatments for a variety of illnesses.

Also of particular interest is a manuscript (the Pennycross Manuscript) signed by a John Beaton (probably signed in the mid-17th century), which is now in the British library, but sets out in Gaelic, the Rule of Health from

Salerno, and mentions Hippocrates, Galen and Avicenna. It was republished in 1911[6] in Gaelic, Latin and English. It notes for example;

> Regimen Sanitatis est Triplex, that is, there are three aspects to the regulation [rule] of health. Conseruatiuum, maintaining a healthy state, Preseruatiuum, that is foreseeing, Reductiuum, that is restoration, as Galen shows.

This is a very modern view of health and its improvement. The Beatons served Scottish Kings from David I to James VI. In spite of this position of influence and learning, the treatments available were very limited, both from a medical point of view and in relation to surgery. Not until the 18th century did more effective treatments and diagnostic techniques become available. By this time the Edinburgh Medical School was pre-eminent in Europe, itself founded by graduates from the University of Leiden in Holland.

The Beatons were famous and highly regarded and there is even a Gaelic rowing-song written in their honour. It is written to James Beaton the great-grandson of the *Ollamh Muileac,* the Mull Doctor, the John Beaton mentioned above.[7]

He is my darling, James
A man of virtue I would desire;
The Beaton's without a doubt.
A sweetheart I'll not deny,
It would be no wonder with me at all,
That man being proud;
You are a kinsman of the Mull Doctor
Who won honour in the field of battle;
A summons came to you from the King,
To say that he was approaching death;
There was of no need of wiles for them,
To be deceiving you there was no substance to them;
If you happen to me in the little hollow,
I would entice you to the hill,
I myself would lay out my plaid under you,
In the watching-house in the sheiling.

This is one of a number of poems written about individual doctors, though not all end in such an enticing way!

Notes

1   Blind Harry, *Wallace*, rev. William Hamilton of Gilbertfield (Edinburgh: Luath Press, 1996).

2   James K. Cameron, *The First Book of Discipline: with Introduction and Commentary* (Edinburgh: Saint Andrew Press, 1972), pp. 130-32S.

3   James A.H. Murray (ed.), *The Complaynt of Scotland*, (Wales: Llanerch Publishers, 1st pub 1872, reprint 1998).

4   John Bannerman, *The Beatons, a Medical Kindred in the Classical Gaelic Tradition*. (Edinburgh: John Donald Publishers Ltd, 1998).

5   Martin Martin, *A Description of the Western Isles of Scotland* (Edinburgh: Birlinn Press, 1999).

6   H. Cameron Gillies, *Regimen Sanitatis. From the Vade Mecum of the Famous MacBeaths, Physicians to the Lords of the Isles and the Kings of Scotland for Several Centuries*. (Glasgow: Alex MacLaren and Sons, 1911).

7   'The Rowing-song', in John MacKenzie, *Sar-obair nam Bard Gaelach*. 4th ed. trans. Hugh Cheape (Edinburgh: 1877) pp. 389–90.

CHAPTER 5

Medicine and health in the age of the Makars

Of eirthly joy it beiris maist degree
Blyithnes in hart, with small possessioun.
                              Robert Henryson[1]

One of the golden ages of Scottish literature was during the 14th and 15th centuries with the poems of the Makars. The range was considerable and those represented here are only a small part of the whole. The ballads, which also grew up around this time, tell stories of love, battles, domestic arrangements and life of the people of Scotland. This chapter begins with one of these great works from John Barbour, *The Bruce*, as it opens an important aspect of quality of life and well-being.

John Barbour

John Barbour's origins are unclear, though it is interesting to note that his father was likely to have been a barber to a famous Scot. Barbers and surgeons were closely related. John Barbour was a clerk at Dunkeld Cathedral in 1355 then moved to the Archdeaconry in Aberdeen. He was fluent in French and may have studied in France or England. The poem with which he is most associated is 'The Bruce' which was written in 1375. He died in 1395, probably in Aberdeen.

'The Bruce'[2]

A! Fredome is a noble thing
Fredome mays man to haiff liking [lets man have pleasure]

Fredome all solace to man giffis
He levys at es that frely levys
A noble hart may haiff nane es
Na ellys nocht that may him ples [or nothing else that pleases him]
Gyff fredome failyhe, for fre liking [for free decision]
Is yharnyt our all other thing. [is longed for above all else][3]

Freedom is an important component of happiness; personal freedom and the ability to act and speak freely, to enjoy living and be part of a free society; freedom to learn and freedom of opportunity. Professor Duncan's translation of the lines which follow emphasise the personal nature of the 'freedom':

He that is a thrall has nothing; all he has is at the disposal of his Lord, who-ever he is. He does not even have as much freedom as free choice to leave or to carry out, that which his heart inclines him to . . . if a man orders his thrall to do something, and at the same time his wife comes to him and asks her due of him, whether he should set aside his Lord's need, pay first what he owes [to his wife] and then do his Lord's command, or leave his wife's [debt] unpaid and do the things that were commanded of him?

Later in the poem, the King rushes north to Inverurie, where he falls ill.

And thar him tuk sik a sekness
That put him to full hard distress
  He forbar bath drynk and mete
His men na medicine couth get
That ever mycht to the king availe
His force gan him halyly faile [his strength failed him completely]
That he mycht nother rid na ga [that he could neither ride nor walk.][4]

Bruce takes time to improve while his men guard him and carry him to safety.

Later on in the poem when Bruce is in Ireland, there is a strange interlude when a laundry woman with the camp followers becomes ill.

> The king has hard a woman cry
> He askyt quhat that wes in hy
> 'it is the laynder, schyr' said ane, [laundry woman]
> 'that hyr child-ill rycht now has tane, [who is in child birth now]
> And mon leve now behind us her, [and we will leave her here behind]
> Tharfor sho makys yone ivill cher' [5] [she is making such a noise]

The King says no, we cannot leave her in pain. There is no man who would not have pity on her. So the whole army is stopped, a tent is put up, other women called and they wait until she delivered and then ride on.

Robert Henrysoun (Henryson) (c1420–c1490)

Henrysoun's background is unclear though he did have links with Dunfermline where he may have been a schoolmaster. He was also a cleric with legal training, and his works show a remarkable range and reflect life in mediaeval Scotland. This poem about the town mouse and the county mouse contrasts their lifestyles and considers quality of life.

'The tale of the Uponlandis Mouse and the Burgess Mouse'

> This rural mouse into the winter-tide
> Had hunger, cauld, and tholit great distress; [suffered]
> The uther mouse that in the burgh can bide
> Was gild-brother and made ane free burgess
> Toll-free als, but custom mair or less [untaxed]
> And freedom had to gae wherever sho list
> Amang the cheese in ark, and meal in kist. [chest][6]

The country mouse is invited to visit her sister in the town and she is shown the sights and the range of food available. She ends the poem with a reflection;

> But I hard say sho passit to her den
> Als warm as wool, suppose it was not great
> Full beinly Stuffit, baith but and ben [comfortably, parlour and kitchen]

> Of beinis and nuttis, peas, rye and wheat
> Whenever sho list, sho had aneuch to eat
> In quiet and ease, withoutin ony dreid
> But to her sisteris feast nae mair sho yeid[7]

She is happy to remain in her own quiet house without worrying, and with enough to eat. And there is a moral to the tale.

> Thy awin fyre, my freind, sa it be bot and gelid [glee]
> It warmis weill, and is worth gold to the
> And Solomon says, gif that thow will reid,
> 'Under the hevin thair can not better be
> Than ay be blyith and leif in honestie' [honestie, quiet]
> Quhairfoir I may conclude be this reason:
> Of eirthly joy it beiris maist degree
> Blyithnes in hart, with small possessioun.[8]

An interesting conclusion, that earthly joy and happiness occurs with peace and with few possessions. This thought will be echoed throughout this book in relation to quality of life.

'The Testament to Cresseid'

In this long poem there are several verses which describe the problems of leprosy.[9]

> This lipper ludge tak for thy burlie bour [leper's lodge, bower]
> And for thy bed tak now ane bunche of stro [straw]
> For waillit wyne and metis thou had tho [choice, food]
> Tak mowlit breid, peirrie and ceder sour [mouldy, perry, cider]
> Bot cop and clapper now is all ago. [Except for, gone]

> My cleir voice and courtlie carolling
> Where I was wont with ladyis for to sing
> Is rauk as ruik, full hideous, hoir and hace [Raucous as a rook, grating, hoarse]

My plesand port, al utheris precelling [Bearing, excelling]
Of lustines I was maist conding [Beauty, to have the most]
Now is deformit the figour of my face
To luik on it na leid now lyking hes [no person has pleasure]
Sowpit in syte, I say with sair siching [sunk, sorrow, sighing]
Ludgeit amang the lipper leid. 'Allace' [lodges, leper folk]

The facial deformity and the effect on his voice are clearly set out.

'Sum Practysis of Medecyne'[10]

There is much in this poem about contemporary medical practice; the apothecary and the surgeon are noted. One verse entitled 'Dia Custrum' is of particular interest:

The ferd feisik is fine, and of ane felloun pryce [fourth, medicine, high]
Gud for haising, and hosting, or heit at the hairt [hoarseness, cough]
Recipe, thre sponfull of the blak spyce
With ane grit gowpene of the gowk fart; [double handful, cuckoo]
The lug of ane lyoun, the guse of ane gryce [goose, sucking pig]
Ane unce of ane oyster poik at the nether parte [stomach]
Annoyntit with nurice doung, for it is rycht nyce [nurse]
Myngit with mysdirt and with mustart [mouse dirt]
Ye may clamp to this cure and ye will mak cost [add to]
Bayth the bellox of ane brok [testicles]
With thre crawis of the cok
The schadow of ane yule stock
Is gud for the host. [cough]

Henryson has two other poems related to health and illness. In 'Ane Prayer for the Pest'[11] he delivers an impassioned plea to God to help, to forgive our sins and to rid us of the plague. He knows that there is no remedy, and the prayer is for help and succour. The second poem is 'In Prais of Aige'.[12] An old man is heard singing with a gay and sweet voice. He does not want to

49

be young as the older he gets the nearer he is to heaven's bliss. He is happy that his youth has gone.

William Dunbar (c1460–?1520)

William Dunbar was known to be Master of Arts, probably at St Andrews, and travelled widely as a Franciscan Novice. He served at the Court of King James IV. He was a European, with links to the developing culture on the continent. One of his best known poems is *'Lament for the Makaris'* which celebrates the great poets of Scotland.

'Lament for the Makaris (when he was seik)'[13]

> In that in heil wes and gladnes
> I am trublit now with great seicknes
> And feblit with infermitie:
> *Timor mortis conturbat me* [the fear of death disturbs me]

He goes through a list of poets and writers who have died; Chaucer, Gower, the Monk of Bury, Sir Hugh of Eglintoun, Heryot and Wynton, Clerk and Affleck, Holland and Barbour, Shir Mungo Lockert of the Leal, Blind Harry, Robert Henrysoun and many others.

The physicians have not helped to save them and indeed they cannot even help themselves.

> In medicine the most practicians
> Lechis, surgeons and phisicians
> Them self frae dead may not supply
> *Timor mortis conturbat me.*[14]

His conclusion is in the final verse:

> Sen for the deid remeid is none
> Best is that we for deid dispone [prepare]
> Eftir our deid that live may we.
> *Timor mortis conturbat me.*[15]

We must prepare for death so that our work will live on.

'Remonstrance to the King'

In this poem Dunbar lists the many 'servitouris and officiaris' the king has.
These include:

> Kirkmen, courtmen, and craftismen fine
> Doctouris in Jure and Medicine
> Divinouris, rethoris, and philosophouris
> Astrologis, artists and oratouris
> Men of arms, and vailyeand knichtis
> And mony other gudlie wichts;

These also include:

> Printouris, paintours and potingaris;[16]

This latter is the apothecary and medical skill is part of the broader advice
to the King and the court.

'On His Heid-ake'

> My hied did yak yester nicht,
> This day to mak that I nae micht
> So sair the magryme dois me menyie [afflict]
> Peirsing my brow as ony ganyie [dart]
> That scant I look may on the licht[17]

This is an excellent description of migraine, with the pain and the aversion
to light.

In another poem, '*To the Merchantis of Edinburgh*'[18]Dunbar describes Edinburgh and the smells.

> May nane pass throw your principall gaittis
> For stink of haddockis and scattis [skates]

The smells preventing people coming into the city and the merchants need to do something about it.

Sir David Lindsay (c1486–c1555)

Sir David Lindsay was born in 1486 on his father's estate in Fife. It is not clear where he was educated but before 1511 he had a place at the Court. After the death of James IV at Flodden in 1513 he became a Gentleman Usher to the infant James V. From 1530 he was one of the King's Heralds, around 1542 received his knighthood and was appointed as Chief Herald and Lyon King of Arms and visited serveral embassies in Brussels, Paris, London and Denmark. As a Herald he saw dramatic spectacles and theatre. The *Satire* was first performed in 1540 at Linlithgow. He died in 1555.

A Satire of the Three Estates ('Ane Pleasant Satyre of the Thrie Estaitis')[19]

The Three Estates are the church, the nobility and the merchant class. Mediciners and physicians are mentioned on several occasions:

> Let some drink ale, and some drink claret wine
> By great doctors of physic I hear say
> That michty drink comforts the dull ingine! [mind]

The play has a fascinating range of characters including, Diligence, King Humanity, Wantonness, Placebo, Lady Sensuality, Flattery, Falset, Deceit, Good Counsel, The Poor Man and John the Common-Weal.

The Poor Man begins his speech:[20]

> Good man, will you give me of your charity
> And I sall declare to you the black verity.

He then sets out the 'Black Truth' of how, when his father died, then his mother died, his goods were taken from him. Though he had cattle and horses and now he has nothing. His goods have been removed by the vicar and the laird. His wife then died and even more of his goods removed, and now his bairns have to beg for food. He has told the black verity, and his misery.

John the Common-Weal of fair Scotland is then introduced to the King, and he is in rags. He is asked why he is so dressed:[21]

> JOHN: Yea sir, that Gars the Common-Weal want clais
> KING: What is the cause the Common-Weal is crookit [lame]
> JOHN: Because the Common-Weal has been owr-lookit
> KING: What gars thee look sa with a dreary heart
> JOHN: Because the Three Estates gangs all backwart

The Common-Weal needs help or they will have to become Border Reivers. The Three Estates debate the issues and eventually call on Good Counsel, and the merchant says:[22]

> MERCHANT: Sit doun and give us your counsel
> How shall we slaik the great murmell [complaint]
> Of poor people, that is weill knawn
> And as the Common-Weal has shawn
> And als we knaw it is the Kingis will
> That good remede be put there-till

After much discussion and debate Good Counsel and Correction provide the solution:[23]

GOOD COUNSEL (to CORRECTION) Or ye depart, Sir, of this region
Give John the Common-Weal a gay garmoun [garment to replace the rags]
Because the Common-Weal has been owrlookit
That is the cause that Common-Weal is crookit
With singular profit he has been sa suppriset [self interest] [Surprisit-oppressed]
That he is baith cauld, nakit and disguiset [ill-clothed]
CORRECTION: As ye have said Father, I am content
Sergeants, give John a new abilyement [Dress]
Of satin, damas or of the velvet fine
And give him a place in our Parliament syne!

53

The Common-Weal has won the day and will have a place in Parliament to speak for those who are poor. This is once again a recurring theme throughout this history, of the social impact on health and well-being. In each time period discussed in the succeeding chapters this issue will be raised emphasising the importance of social determinants to health.

Sir Robert Aytoun 1569–1638)

Aytoun was from Fife and a graduate of St Andrews. He studied civil law at Paris and became an ambassador. He became the court poet to the Queen of James VI, and wrote in Latin, Greek and English. He is buried in Westminster Abbey.

'Upone Tabacco'

> Forsaken of all comforts but these two,
> My faggott and my pipe, I sitt and muse
> On all my crosses, and almost accuse
> The heavens for dealing with me as they do.
> Then hope steps in and with a smyling brow
> Such cheerful expectations doth infuse
> As makes me think ere long I cannot chuse
> But be some Grandie, whatsoever I am now.
> That hopes and dreams are Couzens, both deceive. [deceivers]
> Then make I this conclusion in my mind,
> Its all one thing, both tends unto one scope
> To live upon tabacco and on hope
> The one's but smoake, the other is but wind.[24]

This is another early poem on the dangers of tobacco.

This period of Scottish history showed that the role of the doctor was limited, and that there was little effective therapy available. Doctors, like the Beatons, did have a role in court circles, but they had, as has been noted, little to offer. The major health problems of pestilence, violence and social issues would take time to resolve, and some remain.

Notes

1   Robert Henryson. *Poems and Fables*, ed. H. Harvery Wood, James Thin (Edinburgh: Mercat Press, 1933) p. 16, ll. 56–63.

2   John Barbour. *The Bruce,* ed. and trans, A.A.M. Duncan, (Edinburgh: Cannongate Classics, 1997).

3   Ibid, p. 57, ll. 225–32.

4   Ibid, p. 321, ll. 35–42.

5   Ibid, p. 593, ll. 275–300.

6   Scott, *Penguin Scottish Verse*, p. 116, ll. 5–11.

7   Ibid, p. 123, ll. 1–7.

8   Henryson. *Poems and Fables*, p. 16, ll. 56–63.

9   Robert Crawford and Mick Imlah, (eds.) *The Penguin Book of Scottsh Verse,* 2nd ed. (The Penguin Press, 2000), p. 68.

10 Henryson, *Poems and Fables*, pp. 157–9.

11 Ibid, p. 163.

12 Ibid, p. 185.

13 Scott, *Penguin Scottish Verse*, p. 148, ll. 1–4.

14 Ibid, p. 149, ll. 21–24.

15 Ibid, p. 151, ll. 21–24.

16 Ibid, p. 143, ll. 1–10 and l 16.

17 Ibid, p. 151, ll.1–5.

18 W. Mackay MacKenzie (ed.), *The Poems of William Dunbar*, (London: Faber and Faber Ltd, 1970), p.81.

19 Sir David Lindsay, *A Satire of the Three Estates*, adapted for Tyrone Guthrie's production at the 1948 Edinburgh Festival. Introduction and notes by Matthew McDiarmid (London: Heinmann Educational Books, 1967).

20 Ibid, p. 107, ll. 1401–2.

21 Ibid, p. 125, ll. 1700–1719.

22 Ibid, p. 129, ll. 1769–74.

23 Ibid, p. 159, ll. 2276–2287.

24 Ibid, p. 208, ll. 1–14.

CHAPTER 6

The Age of Enlightenment and the beginning of scientific medicine

Introduction

The 18th century was a time of great change and energy in Scotland. The century began with Scotland as part of the Union of the Crowns in Great Britain – but with a separate parliament; by 1707, there was Union of the Parliaments between Scotland and England.

There were major rebellions and wars which affected Scotland both at home and overseas. The Stuart-led Jacobite rebellions of 1715 and 1745 inspired many literary endeavours, and the songs and poems emerging from these are still powerfully current to this day. The American War of Independence (1775–1783) and the French Revolution (1789–1792) were likewise seminal events which affected Scotland in many ways, cultural and intellectual. *The Rights of Man* by Thomas Paine, begun in 1791, was used by many and imitated by Burns when he penned 'The Rights of Women' which he used for comic purposes to create a new political sensibility. Here Burns shows his depth of awareness of culture and the political scene in Scotland, and it reflects his broader interest in society and health which will be discussed in detail later.

Scotland was a centre of intellectual activity as it embarked on the Enlightenment; a period from the middle to the end of the century, when Scotland led the way internationally in its enlightenment project in philoso-phy, economics, geology, medicine and science. Names such as Adam Smith, David Hume, James Beattie, Dugald Stewart, Frances Hutcheson, Thomas Reid, William Robertson, Lord Kames, William Ferguson, James Hutton, and many more, advanced new ideas in history, the sciences and what today we would call the social sciences. The Enlightenment focussed one of its

56

centres particularly in Edinburgh, and the great house at Newhailes, in Musselburgh just outside Edinburgh, was said to have the best library in Europe. Lord Hailes, the owner, was himself part of the Enlightenment, as an advocate and historian. In architecture there were the Adam brothers, building some of the great houses of Scotland. Scotland had, at the time five universities, which provided much of the focus for debate and discussion of the newest technological and cultural ideas and many of the great names noted above were staff members. School Academies were also springing up, the first in Perth in 1760 followed by others in Dundee, Inverness and numerous others, whose aims were to teach the classics and promote learning. It is from this time that the Knoxian ideal of the primacy of education might be said genuinely to gain critical mass in Scotland

During this time there was the beginning of emigration, some of it in the wake of the battle of Culloden in 1746, and some of it related to the Highland clearances, mainly in the northern counties, linked to the introduction of sheep farming, though the clearances did not gain large momentum until the early nineteeth century. The relics of these migrations can still be seen in the ruined villages and homes across rural Scotland as poignant reminders of this period of Scottish history.

The reformation of the church in Scotland had occurred in the 16th century, but there was still much fluid religious activity with the secession of various groups related to the Patronage Act of 1712 and subsequent Acts, the development of reformed churches, and the ministers of religion being classified as 'New Lichts' or 'Auld Lichts' by the second half of the 18th century; are all reflected in the literature at the time.

Economically there was significant growth in agriculture, and coal, cotton, and iron industries all began to flourish. James Watt, originally from Glasgow, developed the steam engine which transformed the pattern of industrial work. In the financial sector the Bank of Scotland was founded in 1695, the Royal Bank of Scotland in 1727, together with the British Linen Bank in 1746. All this was not without its problems as the failure of the Darien Scheme in the Isthmus of Panama in 1700, and the collapse of the Ayr Bank in 1776 showed. The population grew significantly. For example, the population in Glasgow was 12,500 in 1708, 25,000 in 1750, and 200,000 in 1830. This caused great pressure on housing and other facilities to meet this growth. In Edinburgh the North Bridge was built in 1772 and the New Town in Edinburgh developed, a glorious architectural expansion, which allowed the city to grow a new character and ethos. With such developments in industry, the universities and in population size, Scotland had the potential to burgeon even further, but as will be seen later in the 19th century, not without additional human cost.

One innovative development was the establishment of New Lanark by David Dale in 1786 and which was subsequently taken further by his son-in-law Robert Owen. This cotton mill village set up for the workers, was a new model for industrial growth, which took into account the needs – spiritual and educational – of the workers. The story behind this initiative is rehearsed in a novel *Margaret Maitland* by Margaret Oliphant (1851), which will be discussed subsequently.

Medicine and science were no exception to the change and development of the country. In the early part of the 18th century the centre of medical education in Europe was in Holland, and in particular in Leiden, where Boerhaave, as the leader of the medical school there, and an outstanding teacher, was the key figure. Many Scots students went there to study and this resulted in the initiation of the Edinburgh Medical School in the latter part of the 18th century, which became the most prominent medical school of its time. It was an outstanding centre with William Cullen (1710–1790), in particular, being a teacher par excellence. He introduced, first in Glasgow, then Edinburgh, the teaching of chemistry. When Cullen moved to Edinburgh his chair in Glasgow was taken by Joseph Black (1728–1799) who discovered the gas Carbon Dioxide. Cullen was followed in Edinburgh by Dr James Gregory (1753–1821) who again was an outstanding academic leader and writer. Gregory's name crops up repeatedly in the creative literature of Scotland, from Burns to Scott, and this will be referred to later in subsequent chapters. At the beginning of the 18th century there was knowledge of anatomy, circulation of the blood, childbirth and of some diseases, but treatment was limited. Throughout the century knowledge advanced considerably, and it was an era of the great collectors, Hans Sloane (1660–1753) and the British Museum, and the Hunter brothers (William and John) in London, for example. William Hunter's (1718–1783) very extensive collection of books, paintings, coins, the natural world and human biology, which included butterflies, animals, and human anatomical dissections, came eventually to Glasgow University and John Hunter's (1728–1793) collection was donated to the Royal College of Surgeons of England. Medical education was organised in the universities but there were also numerous private schools and the medical colleges were also involved. The curriculum was loose and the examinations remained in Latin, but not everyone took them; much of the learning was in the form of apprenticeships with no formal qualifications or certification required. Medical societies became an important part of professional education, the first being the medical student society, the Royal Medical Society, established in Edinburgh in 1734.

There were significant advances in some areas, notably in childbirth where London-based William Smellie (1697–1763) wrote a *Treatise on the theory and practice of Midwifery* (1752). He bequeathed his library to the town of Lanark where he was born. William Hunter (1718–1783), from Long Calderwood, East Kilbride, but practising in London, also made major advances and his *Treatise on the Gravid Uterus* (1774) is a magnificently illustrated volume. Infectious disease was a major issue, but it was not until the end of the century on the 14th May 1796 that Edward Jenner used cowpox to vaccinate a boy named James Phipps against smallpox and showed that it was effective. It had an impact on the 19th century but not, however, the 18th century. It is interesting to note that John Hunter (1728–1793), William's brother had Jenner as a pupil while he taught at Charing Cross Hospital. Clinical practice was carried out mainly in general practice and there were few hospitals;[1] Edinburgh Royal Infirmary was founded in 1729, the oldest voluntary hospital in Scotland and Glasgow Royal Infirmary was established in 1794. Mental hospitals also developed at this time, the earliest being in Montrose in 1782. There was no anaesthesia or antisepsis and surgery was of a limited nature. Herbal remedies and a few potions were generally all that was available. William Withering had discovered that the leaves of the Foxglove containing digitalis could help in the treatment of dropsy (due to heart failure) and wrote this up in 1785.

The literature of Scotland in the 18th century contains some of the most iconic figures seen before or since, the most important being Robert Burns (1759–1796). The next several chapters cover a series of authors from the literature of the 18ᵗʰ century: Robert Ferguson (1750–1774), Robert Burns (1759–1796), Tobias Smollett (1721–1771) together with a number of authors whose work is dealt with only briefly and they will be introduced individually as they occur in the text. These writers show Scottish literature reacting against the dynamic background sketched above.

Note

1   See *Building Up on Our Health: The Architecture of Scotland's Historic Hospitals* (n.p.: Historic Scotland, 2010).

CHAPTER 7

Robert Fergusson

'Mang man, wae's heart! We aften find
The brawest drest want peace of mind,
While he that gangs wi ragged coat
Is weel contentit wi his lot.[1]

Robert Fergusson (1750–1774)

Introduction

As you walk down the High Street in Edinburgh you come across a statue on the pavement just outside the Canongate Kirk. It's of Robert Fergusson and is a depiction full of life and energy. He is buried in the churchyard with an inscription by Robert Burns on his gravestone. The story of Fergusson's early death at the age of twenty-four is one of great sadness and some mystery.[2] He was born in Cap and Feather Close near the Royal Mile and attended the Royal High School in Edinburgh and the High School of Dundee. He matriculated at St Andrews University in 1765. When he left St Andrews he returned to Edinburgh in 1768 and decided not to enter any of the professions, he became a copyist like his father, which gave him time to enjoy the social and cultural aspects of Edinburgh, join the clubs and write his poems. He first published a poem in Scots 'The Daft Days' in 1772 and the first edition of his poems appeared in 1773. He had an energetic social life and at times it appears that he was depressed. Near the end of 1774 he suffered a head injury, apparently after falling down some stairs and was admitted, against his will, to Darien House, a mental institution, where a few weeks later he died.[3] He was only 24, and was buried in an unmarked grave in the Canongate Kirkyard.

His influence was significant, and two people in particular ought to be mentioned as affected. The first was Robert Burns who commissioned a memorial stone with an inscription written by the Ayrshire poet:

> No sculptur'd Marble here nor pompous lay
> No stoned urn nor animated bust
> The simple stone directs pale Scotia's way
> To pour her sorrows o'er her dust.[4]

The second important person influenced was Dr Andrew Duncan (1744–1828) who had visited the young poet in Darien House. In time Duncan was a man of considerable influence in Edinburgh. He became involved in numerous medical societies, and assisted several young men, including Sir Henry Raeburn, who painted his portrait. He was affected by Fergusson's death and, partly as a result, persuaded the Royal College of Physicians and others to create a public lunatic asylum in Edinburgh. The Royal Asylum was eventually built in Morningside in 1813.

Fergusson's poems are full of life and excitement and his themes relate to the things around him: the city, the people, their work and pastimes; nature features prominently. He frequently refers to health, quality of life, illness and the role (or otherwise) of the doctor.

Doctors and clinical practice

'Caller [fresh] oysters'[5] (1772)

This poem begins by extolling the quality of the fish from the Firth of Forth and reminds the reader that September is the important month for oysters, 'The halesomest and nicest gear of flesh or fish'. The virtues of oysters are then described, including their capacity to heal and restore:

> O! Then we needna gie a plack [small copper coin]
> For dand'ring mountebank or quack,
> Wha o' their drogs sae bauldly crack, [drugs, boast]
> And spred sic notions,
> As gar their feckless patient tak
> Their stinkin potions.

Come prie, frail man! for gin thou art sick, [taste]
The oyster is a rare cathartic,
As ever doctor patient gart lick
To cure his ails;
Whether you hae the head or heart-ake,
It ay prevails.

Ye tiplers, open a' your poses, [money boxes]
Ye wha are faush'd wi plouky noses!
Fling owr your craig sufficient doses, [throat]
You'll thole a hunder, [tolerate]
To fleg awa your simmer roses, [frighten, skin rash from drink]
And naething under.

Whan big as burns the gutters rin,
Gin ye hae catcht a droukit skin,
To Luckie Middlemist's loup in, [An Inn in the High Street]
And sit fu snug
Owr oysters and a dram o' gin,
Or haddock lug.

Oysters it seems can cure anything, and much better than the pills and potions the doctor can prescribe. They can even remove blemishes from the skin and spots on the nose from overindulgence. Fergusson, as a Tory, was sceptical of progress and wanted to believe in natural life and remedies. He was an idealist and considered the natural way appropriate.

'Caller Water'[6] (1773)

In the same way the way the properties of fresh water are described.

My muse will no gang far frae hame,
Or scour a' airths to hound for fame;
In troth, the jillet ye might blame [flighty woman]
For thinking on't
Wham eithly she can find the theme [easily]
Of aqua font

It's easy to find good things to help you and water is one of these. However it may be called by a strange Latin name (aqua font) and this can confuse the uninitiated:

> This is the name that doctors use
> Their patients' noddles to confuse;
> Wi simples clad in terms abstruse,
> They labour still,
> In kittle words to gar you roose [use difficult words in search of praise]
> Their want o' skill.

Fergusson's subtext is that this is a common part of the medical aura to use long and complex terms, partly to hide the diagnosis or treatment from the patient but also to give the appearance of learning and power; part, again, of his natural outlook. He also rails against complicated medical terminology:

> But we'll hae nae sic clitter-clatter,
> And briefly to expound the matter
> It shall be ca'd good Caller Water,
> Than whilk, I trou,
> Few drogs in doctors' shops are better
> For me or you.

Fergusson is not impressed by such circumlocution in terminology. He wants simply to call it good fresh water, and does so in Scots, a language suitable for such plain speaking.

> Tho' joints are stiff as ony rung, [staff]
> Your pith wi pain be fairly dung, [done in]
> Be you in Caller Water flung
> Out owr the lugs,
> 'Twill mak you souple, swack and young,
> Withouten drugs.

This stanza is one of the most interesting in the poem. With some optimism, it suggests that dipping in water is able to be effective in various illnesses. It might be recalled that Burns was subject to such treatment, which almost certainly hastened his death. The medical literature of the time was encouraging of such methods.

> Tho' cholic or the heart-scad teaze us, [heart burn]
> Or ony inward pain should seize us,
> It masters a' sic fell diseases
> That would ye spulzie, [spoil]
> And brings them to a canny crisis,
> Wi little tulzie. [trouble]

> What makes Auld Reikie's dames sae fair?
> It canna be the halesome air
> But caller burn beyond compare,
> The best of ony,
> That gars them a' sic graces skair, [take fright]
> And blink sae bonny.

The instinct to rely on nature is understandable, but as society was becoming ever more complicated, this could be seen as naïve. There is also a telling reference here to the air quality in Edinburgh in the 18th century which was less than wholesome with the removal of rubbish and excrement a rather limited exercise. Fergusson's poem was written shortly after the new bridge in Edinburgh was built and which was a defining change that would lead to the development of the New Town, where the air would be cleaner in contrast to the Old Town where the smells would remain. Here we begin to see the social divisions which bring about variations in health. Fergusson is also interested in ancient water sources:

> On May-day in a fairy ring,
> We've seen them round St Anthon's spring,
> Frae grass the caller dew draps wring
> To weet their een,
> And water clear as crystal spring,
> To synd them clean. [wash]

The reference here to St Anthon's spring is also relevant. Such healing springs were common in Scotland and will be discussed in more detail in a later chapter.

'To my auld breeks'[7] (1773)

This is a technically well-controlled and riotously funny poem extolling the properties of his old trousers and their importance to the poet. In it, there is reference to the wish to keep well and the role of the doctor's drugs, ineffectual though they are:

> Siclike some weary wight will fill [person]
> His kyte wi drogs frae doctor's bill, [belly]
> Thinking to tack the tither year
> To life, and look baith hale an' fier,
> Till at the lang-run death dirks in,
> To birze his saul ayont his skin. [squeeze]

It's his trousers which have kept him well even though they have holes and are worn, and he is proud of that! Here again Fergusson demonstrates scant confidence in the medicines of the medical profession. There is a humour in the face of the difficulty of the ordinary person easily to control their health. But Fergusson is living at a time just before the Industrial Revolution, when things were to become complex and problematic in terms of health. Such optimism would become outmoded by health issues which could not be faced down in such a manner.

'Braid Claith' [good cloth][8] (1772)

Likewise, speaking of clothes, Fergusson makes the case for being well-dressed in a good suit, in a variety of different settings, especially if you want to do well in society:

> Ye wha are fain to hae your name
> Wrote in the bonny book of fame,

Let merit nae pretension claim
To laurel'd wreath,
But hap ye weel, baith back and wame, [stomach/belly]
In gude Braid Claith.

Like many of Fergusson's poems, with an orthodox 18th century literary theme, he is interested in the gap between appearance and reality. In 'Braid Claith' people assume wholesomeness, wealth and health from the outward appearance. Thus if you are in search of a mate, being well dressed will certainly help in the case of making a successful social union;

For, gin he come wi coat thread-bare,
A feg for him she winna care,
But crook her bonny mou fu sair,
And scald him baith.
Wooers should ay their travel spare
Without Braid Claith.

The doctor has a special need to look good, and can add to his degrees if he has a good set of clothes. This particular reference to what the doctor wears in his or her professional work is picked up later in A.J.Cronin's book *The Citadel*:

Braid Claith lends fock an unco heeze;
Makes mony kail-worms butter-flees;
Gies mony a doctor his degrees
For little skaith:
In short, you may be what you please
Wi gude Braid Claith.

For thof ye had as wise a snout on
As Shakespeare or Sir Isaac Newton,
Your judgment fouk would hae a dout on,
I'll tak my aith,
Till they could see ye wi a suit on
O' gude Braid Claith.

People do make a judgement on you no matter how clever you are. The appearance of the physician and other health professionals may just be important no matter how well qualified they may be. Here Fergusson puts his finger on something that was to become increasingly important in Scotland and elsewhere in the succeeding centuries: the social rank of the physician and surgeon as indicated, amongst other things, by appearance and manners.

Health and diet

Fergusson makes many references to the importance of health and to the relevance of diet. He gives some idea of the range of food available across the different groups in the population. He links these to quality of life, particularly in some cases, and to the concept that wealth does not always lead to happiness.

'The Farmer's Ingle'⁹ (1773)

This poem, inspirational to the later and more famous poem by Burns, the 'Cotters Saturday night' (1786), paints the scene in the farm house of an evening, and the warmth of the fire and the welcome:

> Weel kens the gudewife that the pleughs require
> A heartsome meltith, and refreshing synd
> O' nappy liquor, owr a bleezing fire:
> Sair wark and poortith downa weel be join'd.
> Wi butter'd bannocks now the girdle reiks,
> I' the far nook the bowie briskly reams; [ale barrel]
> The readied kail stand by the chimley cheeks,
> And had the riggin het wi welcome steams,
> Whilk than the daintiest kitchen nicer seems.

In spite of this picture the comment that 'Sair wark and poortith downa weel be join'd' illustrates the difficulties the family face where hard work and poor living seem to co-exist in equal measure.

Frae this lat gentler gabs a lesson lear; [Let those
    who have plenty learn a lesson]
Wad they to labouring lend an eident hand,
They'd rax fell strang upo' the simplest fare, [reach]
Nor find their stamacks ever at a stand.
Fu hale and healthy wad they pass the day,
At night in calmest slumbers dose fu sound,
Nor doctor need their weary life to spae,
Nor drogs their noddle and their sense confound,
Till death slip sleely on, and gie the hindmost wound.

The importance of physical work, simple meals (and not too much overeating) and a good sleep will keep the doctor at bay, until death. The same picture and relationship comes up time and time again: healthy living and contentment. Here we find from Fergusson comment on the determinants of health which pertain down to the present. Fergusson can be somewhat backward-looking in the context of an ever more complicated Scottish society; here he voices some universal wisdom that is rightly reiterated by many writers that follow him. For example in *Sunset Song* (1932) by Lewis Grassic Gibbon the same picture can be found. Health cannot always be equated with wealth, or a full stomach with contentment.

'To the Principal and Professors of the University of St Andrews, on their superb treat to Dr Samuel Johnson'[10] (1773)

This poem is about food, particularly 'Scotch' food, and how it should be served. The occasion was the visit of the famous Dr Johnson to St Andrews at which he commented that oats were a feast in England to cows and horses, and in Scotland to people.[11] The poem sets out what Fergusson would have served. It begins by setting the scene in St Andrews:

St Andrews town may look right gawsy,
Nae grass will grow upon her cawsey,
Nor wa-flow'rs of a yellow dye,
Glowr dowy owr her ruins high,
Sin Samy's head weel pang'd wi lear

Has seen the Alma Mater there:
Regents, my winsome billy boys!
'Bout him you've made an unco noise;
Nae doubt for him your bells wad clink,
To find him upon Eden's brink,
An' a' things nicely set in order,
'Wad kep him on the Fifan border:

Then his comment of Johnson's views on oats (aits)

But hear me, lads! gin I'd been there,
How I wad trimm'd the bill o' fare!
For ne'er sic surly wight as he
Had met wi sic respect frae me.
Mind ye what Sam, the lying loun!
Has in his Dictionar laid doun?
That aits in England are a feast
To cow an' horse an' siccan beast,
While in Scots ground this growth was common
To gust the gab o' man an' woman.

Fergusson's then prepares his own special menu, imaginatively, that he
would like to feed to Dr Johnson:

Imprimis, then, a haggis fat,
Weel tottl'd in a scything pat,
Wi spice and ingans weel ca'd thro',
Had help'd to gust the stirrah's mou,
And plac'd itsel in truncher clean
Before the gilpy's glowrin een.

Secundo, then, a gude sheep's head
Whase hide was singit, never flead,
And four black trotters cled wi girsle,
Bedown his throat had learn'd to hirsle.

What think ye neist, o' gude fat brose
To clag his ribs? a dainty dose!
And white and bloody puddins routh,
To gar the doctor skirl, 'O Drouth!'
Whan he could never houp to merit
A cordial o' reaming claret,
But thraw his nose, and brize and pegh
Owr the contents o' sma ale quegh:
Then let his wisdom girn an' snarl
Owr a weel-toastit girdle farl,
An' learn, that maugre o' his wame,
Ill bairns are ay best heard at hame.
Drummond, lang syne, o' Hawthornden,
The wyliest an' best o' men,
Has gien you dishes ane or mae,
That wad ha' gar'd his grinders play,
Not to roast beef, old England's life,
But to the auld east nook of Fife,
Whare Creilian crafts could weel hae gien
Skate-rumples to hae clear'd his een;
Then neist, whan Samy's heart was faintin,
He'd lang'd for skate to mak him wanton.

A wonderful range of food including 'gude fat brose / to clang to his ribs'. Soup that sticks to the ribs is always a Scottish favourite. What a remarkable choice of food which might certainly have entertained Dr Johnson. In a sense however Fergusson is ramming both food and words down Johnson's throat even as it is true, as Boswell records, that when in Scotland Johnson thoroughly enjoys Scotch broth. Even as Fergusson is culturally defensive in the face of the Englishman, he again points to a considerable truth in commending a simple unpretentious diet.

Social circumstances

Fergusson in many of his poems refers to the social life in the Scottish Capital, engaging with this with some gusto. He gives a good overview of social and cultural mores in Auld Reekie.

'Auld Reekie'[12] (1779)

This poem begins as Edinburgh wakes up. We hear the gossip on the stairs and streets, strangers are recognised and followed to make sure they are up to no badness, and the noise as the schools break at midday. By night the ladies of ill repute ply their wares and there is a good deal of drunkenness. Here we again see Fergusson the conservative who largely believes that human nature in its folly and immorality is essentially unchanging and non-reformable. This is a key issue in the improvement of health for an individual or population.

   There is discussion of death and also drink and snuff, but tobacco is not as yet, a major source of ill health. The scene changes at the weekend as there are visits to church and to the countryside for a change of atmosphere. All in all, the poem gives a strong sense of the minutiae of life in an 18th century town. But Fergusson sees further: he sees poverty and the need to provide more for others. In particular he singles out Provost Drummond and praises his efforts to help the disadvantaged. The reference below to St Mary's is to a wynd in Edinburgh where old clothes are exchanged; Fergusson notes that even poets sometimes need a change of clothes. This part of the poem could be said to be addressed to the Cape Club, of whom Fergusson was a member, as a plea for help. The Cape Club was originally founded in the 1700s and formally constituted in 1764. Its main meeting place was the Isle of Man Arms in the Old Town. All members took a knight's pseudonym when joining, and Fergusson's was 'Sir Precenter'. It had rules and rituals and was composed of a wide variety of members.[13] This is a good early example of an instance of voluntary work, social aid and philanthropic support which were to become such a feature of the 19th century, albeit on a much grander scale:

But chief, O Cape, we crave thy aid,
To get our cares and poortith laid:
Sincerity, and genius true,
Of Knights have ever been the due:
Mirth, music, porter deepest dy'd,
Are never here to worth deny'd;
And health, o' happiness the queen,
Blinks bonny, wi her smile serene.

Now gin a loun should hae his claes
In thread-bare autumn o' their days,
St Mary, brokers' guardian saint,
Will satisfy ilk ail and want;
For mony a hungry writer there
Dives down at night, wi cleeding bare,
And quickly rises to the view
A gentleman, perfite and new.
Ye rich fock, look no wi disdain
Upo' this ancient Brokage Lane!
For naked poets are supplied
With what you to their wants deny'd.

Peace to thy shade, thou wale o' men,
Drummond! relief to poortith's pain:
To thee the greatest bliss we owe,
And tribute's tear shall grateful flow:
The sick are cur'd, the hungry fed,
And dreams of comfort tend their bed:
As lang as Forth weets Lothian's shore,
As lang's on Fife her billows roar,
Sae lang shall ilk whase country's dear,
To thy remembrance gie a tear.
By thee Auld Reikie thrave, and grew
Delightful to her childer's view.
Nae mair shall Glasgow striplings threap [boast]

73

> Their city's beauty and its shape
> While our new city spreads around
> Her bonny wings on fairy ground.

At the end here is a reference to the New Town in Edinburgh, which was just developing. The poem demonstrates some of the social issues and Provost Drummond's help to the poor. The sick are looked after and the hungry fed. Glasgow it seems was doing better, but with the new town, the new City of Edinburgh will also flourish

'An Eclogue'[14] (1773)

The scene is set here at the end of 'An Eclogue' to the coming evening and two farm workers sitting down for a rest before they take the cattle back to town. They draw breath and have a chat:

> 'Twas e'ening whan the spreckled gowdspink sang, [Goldfinch]
> Whan new-faan dew in blobs o' crystal hang;
> Than Will and Sandie thought they'd wrought eneugh,
> And loos'd their sair toil'd owsen frae the pleugh:
> Before they ca'd their cattle to the town,
> The lads to draw their breath e'en sat them down:
> To the stiff sturdy aik they lean'd their backs, [oak bench]
> While honest Sandie thus began the cracks.

Sandie notes that before marriage his wife had been quiet and soft, now her voice is loud and bold. When he arrives home the work is not done, the cheese made or the milking carried out, the fire is not ready and the house not cleaned. To cap it all the gudewife has gone to Edinburgh to get some of her favourite tea. She seems to sit all day with her friends, gossiping and drinking tea:

> Willie
> Her tea! ah! wae betide sic costly gear,
> Or them that ever wad the price o't spier.

Sin my auld gutcher first the warld knew, [grandfather]
Fouk had na fund the Indies, whare it grew.
I mind mysel, it's nae sae lang sin syne,
Whan Auntie Marion did her stamack tyne, [lose her appetite]
That Davs our gardiner came frae Apple-bogg, [an invented place name]
An' gae her tea to tak by way o' drog.

Sandie
Whan ilka herd for cauld his fingers rubs,
An' cakes o' ice are seen upo' the dubbs;
At morning, whan frae pleugh or fauld I come,
I'll see a braw reik rising frae my lum,
An' ablins think to get a rantin blaze
To fley the frost awa an' toast my taes;
But whan I shoot my nose in, ten to ane
If I weelfardly see my ain hearthstane;
She round the ingle with her gimmers sits, [gossips]
Crammin their gabbies wi her nicest bits,
While the gudeman outby maun fill his crap
Frae the milk cogie, or the parritch cap.

The scene of marital bliss recorded here begins to represent the change in the role of women, an aspect of social life which has continued to change since then. The tea-drinking episode is later recorded in *Annals of the Parish*[15] by John Galt as he wrote of this period from the perspective of the early 19th century. Although a small detail of the poem, we see, then, a larger scale shift in society with implications for well-being. It is a hard life for a herd; cold feet and hands that need warming at the fire. His wife and her friends sit talking and gossiping while he has to get his own food. This is a delightful picture of home life.

'The Farmer's Ingle'

This poem has already been noted in relation to the issues of food and a health promoting life. However later in the poem there is a section on family life and the discussion over supper. There is talk particularly of the weather – the showers, the floods and the winter, and about the Kirk and the market. We see, then, co-ordinates of a social scene that if not completely vanished within a few years is only one of many more complex set-ups in society, including the urban scene. In the 'Farmer's Ingle' young love becomes a topic as well as the issue of an illegitimate child and the punishment required: to sit on the cutty-stool and be reprimanded by the minister (Mess John). Burns' 'The Fornicator's Court', sometimes known as 'Libel Summons'[16] takes this even further and describes the social setting of such misdemeanours in more detail. But at least the children in Fergusson's poem are quiet now that they have been fed. Then the stories of witches and warlocks and ghosts begin, linked to the kirk-yard drear:

> The couthy cracks begin when supper's owr,
> The cheering bicker gars them glibly gash
> O' simmers showery blinks and winters sour,
> 'Whose floods did rest their mailings' produce hash:
> 'Bout kirk and market eke their tales age on,
> How Jock woo'd Jenny here to be his bride,
> And there how Marion, for a bastard son,
> Upon' the cutty-stool was forced to ride,
> The woeful scald o' our Mess John to bide.
>
> The fient a cheep's amang the bairnies noo; [scarcely]
> For a' their anger's wi their hunger gane:
> Ay maun the childer, wi a fastin mou,
> Grumble and greet, and make an unco mane,
> In rangles round before the ingle's lowe:
> Frae gudame's mouth auld warld tale they hear,
> O' warlocks louping round the wirrikow,
> O' ghaists that win in glen and kirk-yard drear,
> Whilk touzles a' their tap, and gars them shak wi fear.[17]

Quality of life

This is an important theme in Fergusson's work. It relates mainly to happiness and good relationships with others in a social setting. It also contrasts issues of wealth and poverty and makes the point, which will be discussed later, that you can have good health and quality of life, but not be rich. Perhaps the best introduction to the theme is 'The Daft Days' where Fergusson begins by describing the dark winter nights and that no one can get much pleasure from snowy hills and barren plains. But come into the city, the old town of Edinburgh, which is a snug 'bield', warm and friendly, meet some old friends and have a drink, or even a Highland reel, the best thing to cheer a person up. The New Year is coming and a cause for celebration.

'The Daft Days'[18] (1772)

Auld Reikie! thou'rt the canty hole,
A bield for mony caldrife soul, [shelter, cold]
Wha snugly at thine ingle loll,
Baith warm and couth,
While round they gar the bicker roll [drinking vessel]
To weet their mouth.

When merry Yule-day comes, I trou,
You'll scantlins find a hungry mou; [scarcely]
Sma are our cares, our stamacks fou
O' gusty gear,
And kickshaws, strangers to our view, [delicacies]
Sin fairn-year. [last year]

Ye browster wives, now busk ye braw,
And fling your sorrows far awa;
Then come and gie's the tither blaw
Of reaming ale,
Mair precious than the well of Spa,
Our hearts to heal.

Then, tho' at odds wi a' the warl',
Amang oursels we'll never quarrel;
Tho' Discord gie a canker'd snarl
To spoil our glee,
As lang's there's pith into the barrel
We'll drink and 'gree.

Fidlers, your pins in temper fix,
And roset weel your fiddle-sticks;
But banish vile Italian tricks
Frae out your quorum,
Nor fortes wi pianos mix —
Gie's Tulloch Gorum.

For nought can cheer the heart sae weel
As can a canty Highland reel;
It even vivifies the heel
To skip and dance:
Lifeless is he wha canna feel
Its influence.

Let mirth abound, let social cheer
Invest the dawning of the year;
Let blithesome innocence appear
To crown our joy;
Nor envy wi sarcastic sneer
Our bliss destroy.

And thou, great god of Aqua Vitae
Wha sways the empire of this city,
When fou we're sometimes capernoity, [irritable]
Be thou prepar'd
To hedge us frae that black banditti,
The City Guard.

The New Year has come in and the people are happy in their warm houses and pubs, eating, drinking and dancing. But in the back of their minds they realise that they might become troublesome and the City Guard are there to remind them to behave. These imposers of social order, we are reminded across a number of poems by Fergusson, are bad for the collective peace of the townsfolk. Fergusson's poem is perhaps the mark of one of the last Scottish writers, however, who can write fairly securely about the calendar of the year and a tight-knit population whose particular cultural, social and health problems represent relatively known quantities.

'Hame content'[19]

This poem begins with an interesting message from the 18th century about health promotion:

> Now when the dog-day heats begin
> To birsel and to peel the skin [scorch]
> May I lie streekit at my ease
> Beneath the caller shady trees

The health-related dangers of sunshine are here clearly recognised. The poem then proceeds to consider herds and cottar folk and what matters to them and their health. They are able to wander over hills and rocks without aches or pains, which those with easy lives would not be able to do:

> To Jook the simmer's rigour there,
> And breathe a while the caller air
> 'Mang herds, an' honest cottar fock,
> That till the farm and feed the flock;
> Careless o' mair, wha never fash
> To lade their kist wi' useless cash,
> But thank the gods for what they've sent
> O' health eneugh, and blyth content,
> An' pith, that helps them to stravaig [wander]
> Owr ilka cleugh and ilka craig,

Unkend to a' the weary granes [groans]
That aft arise frae gentler banes,
On easy-chair that pamper'd lie,
Wi banefu viands gustit high, [rich flavoured food]
And turn and fald their weary clay,
To rax and gaunt the live-lang day.

What we have is a plea for early rising and exercise and less thought of filling the kist with money. This text, in particular, is a compendium of the health themes already identified in Fergusson's poetry.

Finally in this section the poem the 'Ode to the Gowdspink'[20] (1773) (the Goldfinch) has a short section which seems to say what Fergusson feels:

'Mang man, wae's heart!we aften find
The brawest drest want peace of mind,
While he that gangs wi ragged coat
Is weel contentit wi his lot.

This poem of Fergusson emphasises again that peace and rest are not in possessions, and that fortunes come with a cost. Freedom is what matters, and without freedom, would I care for life?

Discussion

The health messages in Fergusson's poems are quite clear and remarkably modern. There is no mention of tobacco of course nor drugs, and violence is noted only in passing. But otherwise all the ingredients of a healthy life are recorded; physical activity, a balanced diet, the problems of alcohol abuse and of unprotected sexual activity. There is little mention of fruit and vegetables as a food group and these are certainly not given prominence in the feast for Dr Johnson if he wishes to give the lexicographer a healthy and balanced diet.

His views on doctors are interestingly of their time; medical practitioners have little to contribute and the drugs used are no better than tea, oysters, or fresh water. This view of natural physic was of course justified at this time, or at least was understandable, as the knowledge of disease and health was limited.

Social issues are well described and engaged. The family interactions, husband and wife clashes, and the children needing fed are of course ubiquitous through the ages and are central to communal health. There are some important comments on the poor and their need for special help and care. Fergusson's plea for more help is an important one, and crucial. It reflects the beginning of social concerns about those who are disadvantaged. As one reads the poems there is a strong impression of the dirt and the squalor in ordinary homes, but at the same time the care taken to keep them tidy and clean. There are references to the role of women and the stereotypic roles they played out; the stirrings and gossip over tea make fascinating and informative reading about the social conditions of the day. Women's health is certainly not glimpsed as a specific issue. There is little in the poems on education and its role in improving health.

Perhaps the most difficult issue however relates to the relationship between health and quality of life, and wealth. Fergusson and many other writers during this period make the point that you can be happy and healthy but have little money or possessions. Indeed there is a contrast between those who have and have not, and generally speaking the poorest are the better for it. This remains difficult as the evidence is overwhelming that health status in terms of life expectancy is well correlated with wealth, as is quality of life; generally the poorer the person the poorer the health. This is seen in many cultures and over a long period of time. There is a sentimental attachment to the notion that poor people are superior morally and that the rich are weak and feeble. It sounds good, and the lines are powerful:

>'Mang man, wae's heart! We aften find
>The brawest drest want peace of mind,
>While he that gangs wi ragged coat
>Is weel contentit wi his lot.[21]

But do they stand up to scrutiny? This will be a recurring feature of the 18th century period of Scottish literature. For example in Burns his 'Epistle to Davie, a brother poet' says,

It's no in titles nor in rank
It's no in wealth like Lon'on Bank
　　To purchase peace and rest
It's no in makin muckle mair
Its no in books, its no in lear
　　To mak us truly blest
If happiness hae not her seat
An' centre in the breast
We may be wise or rich or great
　　But never can be blest
　　Nae treasures or pleasures
　　Could make us happy lang
　　The heart ay's the part ay
　　That makes us right or wrang[22]

The inference is the same; wealth, rank and power are not the things which give happiness or health. But is it true? Such a comment can be explained to some extent as emanating from a society where social mobility was rather limited, and such literary tropes perhaps represent a fictional feel good factor. Their effect on health, however, is more uncertain, perhaps not least when we consider the early age at which both Fergusson and Burns died. This is an issue which will be noted as the subsequent literature is explored.

The loss of Fergusson at such a young age, and with so much promise, took away a poet with much to give. His comments on the social fabric of Scotland, and how its people lived and died, are unique.

Notes

1　Robert Fergusson, 'Ode to the Gowdspink' in *Selected Poems*, ed. James Robertson (Edinburgh: Polygon, 2007), p. 162, ll. 21–4.

2　Alexander Grosart, *Robert Fergusson* (Edinburgh: Oliphant, Anderson and Ferrier, 1898) and David Daiches *Robert Fergusson* (Edinburgh: Scottish Academic Press, 1982).

3　Edward Morgan, 'A Scottish Trawl', in Christopher Whyte, *Gendering the Nation: Studies in Modern Scottish Literature* (Edinburgh: Edinburgh University Press, 1995), pp. 208–10.

4 'Letter from Robert Burns to the Bailies of the Canongate, 6 February 1787', in Maurice Lindsay, *The Burns Encyclopedia* (New York: Robert Hale, 1980), p. 131.

5 'Caller Oysters' in Fergusson, *Selected Poems*, pp. 65–9.

6 'Caller Water' in Fergusson, *Selected Poems*, pp. 98–101.

7 'To my auld breeks' in Fergusson, *Selected Poems*, pp. 189–192.

8 'Braid Claith' in Fergusson, *Selected Poems*, pp. 77–9.

9 'The Farmer's Ingle' in Fergusson, *Selected Poems*, pp. 130–4.

10 'To the Principal and Professors of the University of St Andrews, on their superb treat to Dr Samuel Johnson', in Fergusson, *Selected Poems*, pp. 165–8.

11 Dr Johnston in *Dictionary of the English Language* (1775), in *The Oxford Dictionary of Quotations*, 3rd ed. (Oxford: Oxford University Press, 1980), p. 281.

12 'Auld Reekie', in Fergusson, *Selected Poems*, pp. 102–115.

13 R. Chambers, *The Traditions of Edinburgh* (Edinburgh: W.R. Chambers, 1868), pp. 164–5.

14 'An eclogue', in Fergusson, *Selected Poems*, pp. 84–88.

15 John Galt, *Annals of the Parish* (Oxford: Oxford University Press, 1989), pp. 12–13.

16 Robert Burns, 'Libel Summons', in *The Complete Poetical Works of Robert Burns*, pp. 227–230.

17 Robert Fergusson, *Selected Poems*.

18 'The Daft Days', in Fergusson, *Selected Poems*, pp. 52–4.

19 'Hame content', in Fergusson, *Selected Poems*, pp. 149–53.

20 'Ode to the Gowdspink', in Fergusson,, *Selected Poems*, pp. 162–4.

21 'Ode to the Gowdspink', in Fergusson, *Selected Poems*, p. 162, ll. 21–24.

22 'Epistle to Davie, a brother poet', in *The Complete Poetical Works of Robert Burns*, p. 87, ll. 57–70.

CHAPTER 8

Robert Burns, remember
Tam o' Shanter's mare

Now, wha this tale o truth shall read,
Ilk man, and mother's son, take heed:
Whene'er to drink you are inclin'd,
Or cutty sarks rin in your mind,
Think! Ye may buy the joys o'er dear:
Remember Tam o' Shanter's mare.[1]

Robert Burns

Introduction

Robert Burns (1759–1796) is an iconic figure in Scottish literature. Born in a cottage in Alloway on the 25th of January 1759, his poems and songs reflect Scotland as it was on the cusp of great change, and provide an insight into the public knowledge of health and medicine at the time. The context is the Enlightenment in Scotland, and Burns was well connected to many of the important figures of this milieu, including prominent medical men, and certainly knew of them. He was a person of wide reading and contacts. The main source for this chapter came from the poems themselves, supplemented with several reference sources including, *The Letters of Robert Burns*; *Robert Burns and Mrs Dunlop: Correspondence now published in full*; *Robert Burns and the Medical Profession* and *William Maxwell to Robert Burns*.[2]

Burns would have been familiar with traditional medicine of the time and had access to contemporary books on health. For example it is worth noting at this stage his reference in 'Death and Doctor Hornbook' (1787) to a very popular medical book of the time, *Buchan's Domestic Medicine* (William Buchan 1729–1805)[3] meant for use in the home;

Ye ken Jock Hornbook i the clachan?
Deil mak his king's-hood in a spleuchan! —
He's grown sae weel acquaint wi *Buchan*
And ither chaps,
The weans haud out their fingers laughin,
An pouk my hips.[4]

The poem suggests that he might have seen other 'medical' books by 'ither chaps.' The reference to Buchan's book is significant. As Bynum and Porter point out that *Domestic Medicine* was an attempt, set out in the Preface of 1769, to educate the poor on health matters and to warn against the indiscriminate use of herbs and unqualified practitioners. It also made the point that those ladies and gentlemen who lived in the country had a responsibility to teach the poor about health and sickness.[5] It is interesting to note that in the later editions of the book (for example the 1824 edition) this has changed in tone, and, just as relevant, there is a new section on the use of sea-bathing and its value in health care, perhaps a contributory factor in advancing the illness of the poet himself. Buchan notes, 'A great advantage of sea-water in chronic diseases is that it may be persevered in for a long time, without weakening the intestines or the constitution.'[6] Burns' poems range over many different health-related subjects from prevention and early diagnosis to death and its impact. There are poems which reflect the lifestyle determinants of health (eating and drinking), and major topics such as poverty, old age and their consequences. He discusses doctors and their ineffectiveness, and the importance of learning. There are a considerable number of references to quality of life and happiness, and what they mean and, like Fergusson, Burns contrasts the poor honest workman with the rich knights and lords. For those who recognise the political nature of the delivery of a health service, they might try to answer his question posed in 'The Fete Champetre' (1834) where the of the Member of Parliament who is sent to the House of Commons (St Stephen's House) by the voters, is to determine health policy, and to do the errands (the wishes) of the people. The narrator asks:

O, wha will to Saint Stephen's House,
To do our errands there, man?

> O, wha will to Saint Stephen's House
> O, th' merry lads of Ayr, man?
> Or will ye send a man of law?
> Or will ye send a sodger?
> Or him wha led o'er Scotland a'
> The meikle Ursa-Major?[7]

Who does represent us in Parliament (St Stephen's House) and to which Parliament would it now refer!

This chapter reviews these topics and relates the poems to both 18[th]century health issues and approaches to care, and to those of the 21[st]century.

Prevention and early diagnosis

In Burns' poem 'Address to the unco guid, or the rigidly righteous' (1787) he sets out a very modern view of the problems of developing a habit of drinking to excess, as discussed in the introduction:

> See Social Life and Glee sit down
> All joyous and unthinking,
> Till, quite transmugrify'd, they're grown
> Debauchery and drinking:
> O, would they stay to calculate
> Th' eternal consequences,
> Or your more dreaded hell to state –
> Damnation of expenses![8]

Excessive alcohol comsumption begins with a few drinks and social mixing until it descends into debauchery. If people would just think of the consequences, of the effects of such habits surely they wouldn't go to excess. Many of the current public health messages reflect the same outcome. It would be surprising if those who smoke in this country in the 21st century were not aware of the dangers, yet twenty per cent of adults were recorded as still smoking in 2010.[9] Burns follows this with an even more interesting comment, trying to answer this question he enjoins:

> Then gently scan your brother man,
> Still gentler sister woman;
> Tho they may gang a kenning wrang,
> To step aside is human:
> One point must still be greatly dark,
> The moving Why they do it;
> And just as lamely can ye mark,
> How far perhaps they rue it.

Such behaviour is a human failing, and there is no simple answer as to why they do it. Just as importantly they are likely to rue it, and this applies equally to men and women. The mechanism is the subject of many contemporary research projects in the social sciences.

Perhaps some of Burns' most quoted lines fit in well here from 'To A Louse' (1786):

> O wad some Power the giftie gie us,
> To see oursels as ithers see us!
> It wad frae monie a blunder free us
> An foolish notion[10]

When it comes to early diagnosis and prevention, Burns is again remarkably positive in a quotation from 'Death and Dr Hornbook'. In this poem, which will be referred to in more detail later, Burns sets out the qualities of a local 'quack' and in this section he informs us how the 'doctor' can even make a diagnosis at a distance, without ever having seen the patient. He describes, with great accuracy, the current method of large bowel cancer screening, though the language would not necessarily be used in any public information campaign:

> Ev'n them he canna get attended,
> Altho their face he ne'er had kend it,
> Just shite in a kail-blade, an send it,
> As soon's he smells 't,
> Baith their disease, and what will mend it,
> At once he tells 't.

Here is a simple diagnostic test which allows treatment to be prescribed, at a distance, the forerunner of internet-based testing. Perhaps more interestingly is his final reflection in 'Tam o' Shanter' (1791), used in the introduction to this chapter, where the guid wife summarises the problem and gives clear and unambiguous advice, to young and old:

> Now, wha this tale o truth shall read,
> Ilk man, and mother's son, take heed:
> Whene'er to drink you are inclin'd,
> Or cutty sarks rin in your mind,
> Think! Ye may buy the joys o'er dear:
> Remember Tam o' Shanter's mare.[11]

Burns makes no mention in his poems of smallpox and the development of inoculation as a preventative measure. Smallpox was one of the most prevalent infectious diseases at the time and it perhaps surprising that there is no reference to it in his writings. Evidence that he knew about the procedure for inoculation comes from several of the letters between him and Mrs Dunlop. On four occasions (Letters 25th January 1790, 25th March 1791, 6th April 1791, and 30th April 1791) inoculation and smallpox are mentioned. Burns replies on several occasions. On the 25th of January 1790 he writes to Mrs Dunlop, 'I am every day expecting the doctor to give your little godson [his second son Francis] the smallpox. They are rife in the country, and I tremble for his fate.'[12] Again on the 17th February 1791 he writes:

> As to the little fellow, he is, partiality apart, the finest boy I have long time seen. He is now seventeen months old, has the smallpox and measles over, has cut several teeth, and has never yet had a grain of doctor's drugs in his bowels.[13]

Finally, on the 11th April 1791 he again writes to Mrs Dunlop, 'Do let me hear, by first post, how *cher petit Monsieur* comes on with small pox.'[14] These comments are of some interest for several reasons. First, Dr Edward Jenner from Gloucester is credited with the discovery of vaccination when he inoculated the boy James Phipps on the 14th May 1796, from the hand of a dairy maid who had cowpox. The inoculations referred to in Mrs Dunlop's letter comment on the use of smallpox itself as the agent used, and a quite different and dangerous method of prevention. The second interesting link is that Anne Hunter, a correspondent with Burns, who was married to John Hunter (1728–1793), an old colleague of Jenner's and who famously wrote to him saying, 'But why think. Why not trie the expt' (2nd August 1775, letter in possession of the Royal College of Surgeons of England).[15] Thirdly, there is a whole chapter on smallpox in Buchan, though in the early editions there is no mention of vaccination. In the later editions vaccination (the cowpox method) is treated as a separate subject, and one which is admired by Buchan. Finally, Buchan and Burns shared the same printer, William Creech, in the earlier editions and this may have alerted Burns to Buchan's work.

Robert Burns and the Statistical Account of Scotland

It is of interest to note that Burns was familiar with Sir John Sinclair's work on Scottish Statistics, gathered from parishes across Scotland. Sir John Sinclair (1754–1835) was born in Thurso and had a remarkable career which included agricultural reform. He was the first person to use the term statistics, and to carry out this work on such a grand scale. *The Statistical Account of Scotland* was published in 21 volumes between 1791 and 1799 and was a major step forward in recording and planning communities and nations. Burns was clearly familiar with the work, though not completed in his lifetime, and he comments on some of the findings, for example in a letter to Mr Thomson 7th April 1793. Burns refers to Sir J Sinclair's *Statistical Volumes* in which he picks up a comment as to whether Aberdeen or Ayrshire has the honour of originating the song 'The Lass o' Patie's Mill.

In an undated letter, he writes directly to Sir John Sinclair about:

. . .an issue omitted in the Statistical Account transmitted to you of the parish of Dunscore in Nithsdale. I beg leave to send it to you, because it is new, and may be useful . . . .To store the minds of the lower classes with useful knowledge is certainly of very great importance, both to them as individuals, and to society at large. Giving them a turn for reading and reflection, is giving them a source of innocent and laudable amusement; and besides, raises them to a more dignified degree in the scale of rationality. Impressed with this grand idea, a gentleman in this parish, Robert Riddell, Esq, of Glenriddell, set on foot a species of circulating library, on a plan so simple as to be practicable in any corner of the country. . . . Mr Riddell got a number of his own tenants, and farming neighbours, to form themselves into a society for the purpose of having a library among themselves . . . Each member, at his entry, paid five shillings; and at each of their meetings, which were held every fourth Saturday, sixpence more . . . At the breaking up of the society . . . they had collected upwards of one hundred and fifty volumes[16]

The significance of this is in Burns' knowledge of the Statistical Account and his wider interest in the culture and history of Scotland. He was interested in people and their lives and was sufficiently aware to write and to challenge those in authority. This awareness of current issues in politics, health, cultural and social circumstances is a defining feature of Burns' writing

Drink

As a subject, the consumption of alcohol crops up regularly. In the poem 'Scotch Drink' (1786)[17] he sets out its properties.

> On thee aft Scotland chows her cood,
> In souple scones, the wale o food!
> Or tumbling in the boiling flood
> Wi kail an beef:
> But when thou pours thy strong heart's blood
> There thou shines chief
>
> Food fills the wame, an keeps us livin;
> Tho life's a gift no worth receiving,
> When heavy-dragg'd wi pine an grieving;
> But oil'd by thee,
> The wheels o life gae down-hill, scrievin,
> Wi rattling glee.

Robert Burns, remember Tam o' Shanter's mare

> Thee, Ferintosh! O sadly lost!
> Scotland lament frae coast to coast!
> Now colic grips, an barkin hoast
> May kill us a';
> For loyal Forbes' charter'd boast
> Is taen awa!

Food, though it fills us up is not quite enough, we need drink, and Scotch whisky at that and as an extra fillip to the soul as well as the body. The final reference to Ferintosh relates to the problem faced by Forbes of Culloden, when the Westminster Parliament began to tax the whisky made in the Black Isle (Ferintosh). The consequence is that colic and the 'hoast' (the cough) will now go untreated without the use of whisky. Thus the role of government in fiscal policy related to alcohol, tobacco and food cost, can have both a positive and negative impact on health. In the example above, putting the cost of whisky up, means that coughs may not be treated properly.

In the 'Twa Dogs'[18] Burns makes a reference to the means by which drink can take us away from our own troubles and place them elsewhere: 'the Kirk and State', the contemporary issues of patronage and priests, and the eternal issue of taxation. The value of alcohol in easing our existence is set out:

> An whyles twalpennie worth o nappy
> Can mak the bodies unco happy:
> They lay aside their private cares,
> To mind the Kirk and State affairs;
> They'll talk o patronage and priests,
> Wi kindling fury i' their breasts,
> Or tell what new taxation's comin,
> An ferlie at the folk in Lon'on

The issues of alcohol abuse and its management remain high in the political agenda at the start of the 21st century, and Scotland it seems has a particular problem with its control.

Food and diet

Both food and diet are recurring themes in the poems. Sometimes, as in 'A Cotter's Saturday Night' (1786)[19] the text reflects the food as served in the home, albeit here on a special occasion:

> But now the supper crowns their simple board,
> The halesome parritch, chief o Scotia's food;
> The soupe their only hawkie does afford,
> That, 'yont the hallan snugly chows her cood:
> The dame brings forth, in complimental mood,
> To grace the lad, her weel-hain'd kebbuck, fell;
> And aft he's prest, and aft he ca's it guid:
> The frugal wifie, garrulous, will tell,
> How 'twas a towmond auld, sin lint was i' the bell.

Porridge, soup and cheese are served up to impress the young man.

At other times Burns focusses on special delicacies as in 'Address to the Haggis' (1787) on the offal delicacy:

> Fair fa' your honest, sonsie face,
> Great chieftain o the puddin'-race!
> Aboon them a' ye tak your place.
> Painch, tripe, or thairm:
> Weel are ye wordy of a grace
> As lang's my arm.
>
> The groaning trencher there ye fill,
> Your hurdies like a distant hill
> Your pin wad help to mend a mill
> In time o need
> While thro your pores the dews distil
> Like amber bead.[20]

This is, of course in contrast to foreign food:

Robert Burns, remember Tam o' Shanter's mare

Is there that owre his French ragout,
Or olio that wad staw a sow,
Or fricassee wad mak her spew
Wi perfect scunner,
Looks down wi sneering, scornfu view
On sic a dinner?

This is not just a xenophobic comment about foreign food, but is about the virtue of homely simplicity which is preferable to 'luxury'.

Another example of plain food is in 'The Shepherd's Wife'[21] (1796) and the supper expected when the man (the shepherd) gets home:

What will I get to my supper,
Gin I come hame, gin I come hame?
What will I get to my supper,
Gin I come hame again e'en, jo?

Ye'se get a panfu o plumpin parridge,
And butter in them, and butter in them,
Ye'se get a panfu o plumpin parridge,
Gin ye'll come hame again e'en, jo.

A reekin fat hen, weel fryth'd i' the pan,
Gin ye'll come hame, gin ye'll come hame,
A reekin fat hen weel fryth'd i' the pan,
Gin ye'll come hame again e'en jo.

One can almost hear the fat frying and the plump hen cooking. In 21st century terms, perhaps not the best for health.

As with alcohol, diet and the issue of obesity remain a significant problem in Scotland. In the 18th century a greater proportion of the population lived and worked on the land. The diet was mixed, porridge, potatoes, fish, and some meat. It was those who were rich who were the ones with obesity, with rich food, and less exercise. This theme recurs throughout the literature of

Scotland, and the balance between exercise, overeating and the type of food eaten, remains the same today.

Medicine and doctors

Burns' fame and personality took him into contact with many of the doctors in Scotland at the time and there are a number of references to doctors and to clinical practice in his work. Dr William Findlay's erudite work *Robert Burns and the Medical Profession* published by Alexander Gardner, Paisley and London, 1898, summarises some of these links.[22] Appendix 1 provides further information on those doctors who were of significance to the poet's life and work.

Proponents of 'Evidenced-Based Medicine' will be delighted to agree with Burns in his two lines in 'A Dream' (1786): 'But facts are chiels that winna ding, / An downa be disputed'.[23] He had some knowledge of the Edinburgh Medical School as his reference to 'ten Monroes' shows in 'To Robert Graham of Fintry'. The Monroes were a three generation family of anatomists in Edinburgh skilled in dissection. The satire is partly simple comedy but also exposes the fame of Edinburgh medicine!

> Critics – appall'd, I venture on the name;
> Those cut-throat bandits in the paths of fame;
> Bloody dissectors, worse than ten Monroes;
> He hacks to teach, they mangle to expose.[24]

The most obvious reference to doctors is in 'Death and Doctor Hornbook'. Dr Hornbook is a caricature of a local quack, based on a schoolteacher, John Wilson, who dabbled in medicine. Wilson was a Glasgow Graduate and who taught first at Craigie in Ayrshire and in 1781 was appointed schoolmaster in Tarbolton. Burns sets out his competence:

> See, here's a scythe, an there's a dart.
> They hae pierc'd monie a gallant heart;
> But Doctor Hornbook wi his art
> An cursed skill,

Robert Burns, remember Tam o' Shanter's mare

Has made them baith no worth a fart,
Damn'd haet they'll kill!

In summary he is not very competent and has limited skill. Burns follows this up with an exposition of the doctor's armamentarium, and Latin jargon to impress his patients:

And then a' doctor's saws and whittles,
Of a' dimensions, shapes and mettles,
A' kinds of boxes, mugs, and bottles,
He's sure to hae;
Their Latin names as fast he rattles
As A B C.'

'Calces o fossils, earths and trees;
True sal-marinum o the seas:
The farina of beans an pease,
He has't in plenty;
Aqua-fontis, what you please,
He can content ye.'

'Forbye some new, uncommon weapons,
Urinus spiritus of capons;
Or mite-horn shavings, filings, scrapings,
Distill'd per se;
Sal-alkali o midge-tail clippings,
And monie mae.

Hornbook has all the language and the pills, but is still fairly ineffective and he says he can make you feel better. The contents of the shop, interestingly, link back to Henrysoun's '*Sum Practysis of Medicyne*' in Chapter 4, p49 and are similar to the one in Mantua (*Romeo and Juliet*, Act V Scene 1)[25] :

I do remember an apothecary. . .
And in his needy shop a tortoise hung

95

An alligator stuffed and other skins
Of ill-shaped fishes; and about his shelves
A begarrly account of empty boxes
Green earthen pots, bladders and musty seeds
Remnants of packthread, and old cakes of roses

And the final indictment of Burns' is on the quality of Hornbook's clinical practice:

That's just a swatch o Hornbook's way
Thus goes he on from day to day
Thus does he poison, kill, an slay,
An's weel paid for't;
Yet stop me o my lawfu prey,
Wi his damn'd dirt.

Hornbook is well paid, indeed that may be his primary motivation, but has little to offer. Even though he knows his therapy is ineffective, he continues to treat those who seek his advice. Dr Hornbook's ability to diagnose and treat from a distance has already been referred to.

In another reference to diagnostic techniques, he refers in the 'Epistle to John Goldie, in Kilmarnock' (1785), to the testing of water, a reference to urinary testing:

Poor gapin, glowerin Superstition!
Wae's me, she's in a sad condition!
Fye!, bring Black Jock, her state physician,
To see her water!
Alas! There's ground for great suspicion
She'll ne'er get better.

Enthusiasm's past redemption
Gane in a gallopin consumption:
Not a' her quacks, wi' a their gumption.
Can ever mend her;

Her feeble pulse gies strong presumption,
She'll soon surrender.[26]

The 'Black Jock' referred to is the Reverend John Russell an 'Auld Licht' minister with whom Burns disagreed theologically. There is an interesting reference here to a 'feeble pulse' and Burns' own condition following rheumatic fever with its effect on the heart would have made him aware of this symptom. The testing of urine was limited to the colour, which might give some indication of a diagnosis, or to the taste, a standard method of diagnosing sugar in the urine. The pisspot being examined was a common way of depicting the physician.

Burns also knew many doctors, in Edinburgh and in Ayrshire and Dumfries. In his own illnesses, a broken ankle, and in his, most probably, rheumatic fever for example, he had direct knowledge of them. His own doctor in his last illness (Dr Maxwell) is the subject of a short poem, recorded in a letter to Mr Thomson, September 1794. Burns writes:

How do you like the following epigram, which I wrote the other day on a lovely young girl's recovery from a fever? Dr Maxwell was the physician, who seemingly saved her from the grave; and to him I address the following.

Maxwell, if merit here you crave
That merit I deny;
You save fair Jessie from the grave!
An angel could not die![27]

The key to this epigram is that Dr Maxwell 'seemingly' saved her, but she was so fair she could not die, and Maxwell should not get the credit.

Illness

References to illness and old age reflect the medical practice of the times. But even here Burns is remarkably modern, with his thoughts on psychosomatic illness. In 'The Twa Dogs' one of the canines notes:

Lord, man, were ye but whyles whare I am,
The gentles, ye wad ne'er envy 'em!
It's true, they need na starve or sweat,
Thro winter's cauld, or simmer's heat:
They've nae sair wark to craze their banes,
An fill auld age wi grips and granes;
But human bodies are sic fools,
For a' their colleges an schools,
That when nae real ills perplex them,
They mak enow themsels to vex them;
An aye the less they hae to sturt them,
In like proportion, less will hurt them.
A countra fellow at the pleugh,
His acre's till'd, he's right enough;
A countra girl at her wheel,
Her dizzen's dune, she's unco weel;
But gentlemen, an ladies warst,
Wi' ev'n down want o wark are curst.
They loiter, lounging, lank an lazy:
Tho deil-haet ails them, yet uneasy:
Their days insipid, dull an tasteless;
Their nights unquiet, lang an restless.

Again we find the comparison between rich and poor, and the way in which ladies and gentlemen are uneasy and restless, while the poor have no time to manufacture ill health. Health is much more than a series of symptoms or a disease, it relates to the whole person; physical, mental, social and spiritual. The key lines however must be:

But human bodies are such fools
For a' their colleges and schools
That when nae real ills perplex them
They make enow themsels to vex them

What insight into human behaviour. Burns instinctively notes that we can become ill when there is nothing wrong, in spite of our knowledge and intelligence.

The 'Address to the toothache' (1794) is a classic, but covers more than just the teeth. Burns notes in a letter to William Creech on 30th May 1789, his personal experiences:

> I had intended to have troubled you with a long letter, but at present the delightful sensations of an omnipotent Toothache so engross all my inner man, as to put it out of my power even to write nonsense. . . .while fifty troops of infernal spirits are driving post from ear to ear along my jaw bones.[28]

> My curse upon your venom'd stang,
> That shoots my tortur'd gums alang,
> An thro my lug gies monie a twang
> Wi gnawing vengeance,
> Tearing my nerves wi bitter pang,
> Like racking engines!
>
> A' down my beard the slavers trickle,
> I throw the wee stools o'er the mickle,
> While round the fire the giglets keckle,
> To see me loup,
> And raving mad, I wish a heckle
> Were i' their doup
>
> When fevers burn, or ague freezes,
> Rheumatics gnaw, or colic squeezes,
> Our neebors sympathise to ease us,
> Wi pitying moan;
> But thee! – thou hell o a' diseases –
> They mock our groan!'[29]

The reference to 'ague' is of interest. It is a term not used nowadays, and refers to a fever, recurring every three or four days (tertian or quartan) generally covering any illness, such as typhus, enteric fevers or malaria. There is evidence that malaria occurred in Scotland, especially in marshy areas, and the mosquito vector is still present. The elimination of malaria was due to several factors, the drainage of swampy ground, the introduction of root crops, improved housing and removal of damp dark places and insecticides. The standard treatment at the time was Peruvian bark (Cinchona) whose active ingredient is quinine. In Buchan's *Domestic Medicine* (1824 edition), there is a whole section in 'Intermittent Fevers and Ague' and includes the use of the Peruvian bark. With climate change occurring and a warmer atmosphere present, the possibility of ague recurring should be considered![30]

Abortion is another subject that is dealt with in a poem called 'The Fornicator's Court', or sometimes called 'Libel Summons' or 'The Court of Equity' and also mentioned with dark humour in 'Death and Dr Hornbook'. The narrator/court member reveals that:

> First, You, John Brown, there's witness borne,
> And affidavit made and sworn,
> That ye hae bred a hurly-burly
> 'Bout Jeany Mitchel's tirlie-whirlie
> And blooster'd at her regulator,
> Till a' her wheels gang clitter-clatter.
> And farther still, ye cruel Vandal,
> A tale might even in hell be scandal!
> That ye hae made repeated trials
> Wi drugs and draps in doctor's phials,
> Mixt, as ye thought, wi fell infusion,
> Your ain begotten wean to poosion.
> And yet ye are sae scant o grace,
> Ye daur to lift your brazen face
> And offer for to take your aith,
> Ye never lifted Jeany's claith.-
> But tho ye should yoursel manswear,
> Laird Wilson's sclates can witness bear.
> Ae e'ening of a Mauchline fair,

That Jeany's masts they saw them bare;
For ye had furl'd up her sails,
And was at play – at heads and tails.[31]

The details given in this poem suggest that procuring an abortion was common knowledge and that process of abortion, no matter how offensive and frowned on it might be, was a recognised procedure.

Old age is beautifully covered by Burns, perhaps especially in 'John Anderson, My Jo'.[32] Here the life long relationship between a man and wife is described with a picture painted in words straddling the aging process; the change from young to old, but the retention of the love between them:

> John Anderson my jo, John,
> When we were first acquent,
> Your locks were like the raven,
> Your bonie brow was brent;
> But now your brow is beld, John,
> Your locks are like the snaw,
> But blessings on your frosty pow,
> John Anderson, my jo!
>
> John Anderson my jo, John,
> We clamb the hill thegither,
> And monie a cantie day, John,
> We've had wi ane anither;
> Now we maun totter down, John,
> And hand in hand we'll go,
> And sleep thegither at the foot,
> John Anderson my jo!

The problems of old age are also recorded in 'What can a young lassie do wi' an auld man' (1792). We are told of him:

> He's always compleenin frae morning to eenin;
> He hoasts and he hirples the weary day lang;

101

He's doylt and he's dozin, his blude it is frozen —
O, dreary's the night wi a crazy auld man![33]

Death of course was the poor man's friend, and this is noted in 'Man was made to Mourn' (1786). It links poverty to death:

> See yonder poor, o'erlabour'd wight,
> So abject, mean, and vile,
> Who begs a brother of the earth
> To give him leave to toil;
> And see his lordly fellow-worm
> The poor petition spurn,
> Unmindful, tho a weeping wife
> And helpless offspring mourn.[34]

And death comes as a relief:

> O Death! The poor man's dearest friend,
> The kindest and the best!
> Welcome the hour my aged limbs
> Are laid with thee at rest!
> The great, the wealthy fear thy blow,
> From pomp and pleasure torn;
> But oh! A blest relief for those
> That weary-laden mourn!

In 'Tam Sampson's Elegy' (1787) similar sentiments are expressed:

> In vain auld age his body batters,
> In vain the gout his ancles fetters,
> In vain the burns cam down like waters,
> An acre braid!
> Now ev'ry auld wife, greetin, clatters:
> 'Tam Samson's dead![35]

The reference to a battered body, gout, and urine dribbling out related to prostatic hypertrophy ('burns cam down like waters') is a remarkably good picture of old age.

Death was common, and within families it would not be unusual to lose one, or several, children. A glance at the tombstones in any old kirkyard will confirm that. It was familiar, and at the same time released people, especially the poor from misery. Palliative care, as a speciality, was not available and medical help limited in terms of drugs for pain relief, relief of breathing difficulties, nausea, loss of appetite and weight loss.

Burns makes a number of comments on his own medical conditions own illness. For example in relation to depression he writes to Mr Cunningham 25th February 1794:

Canst thou minister to a mind diseased? Canst thou speak peace and rest to a soul tossed on a sea of troubles, without one friendly star to guide her course, and dreading that the next surge may overwhelm her? Canst thou give to a frame, trembling alive as the tortures of suspense, the stability and hardihood of the rock that braves the blast? If thou canst not do the least of these, why wouldst thou disturb me in my miseries with thy inquiries about me?

For these two months I have not been able to lift a pen. My constitution and frame were, *ab origine* blasted with a deep incurable taint of hypochondria, which poisons my existence. Of late a number of domestic vexations, and some pecuniary share in the ruin of these ****** times; losses which though trifling, were yet what I could ill bear, have so irritated me that my feelings at times could only be envied by a reprobate spirit listening to the sentence that doomed it to perdition.

Are you deep in the language of consolation? I have exhausted in reflexion every topic of comfort . . . . Still there are two great pillars that bear us up, amid the wreck of misfortune and misery. The one is composed of the different modifications of a certain noble, stubborn something in man, known by the names of courage, fortitude, magnanimity. The other is made up of those feelings and sentiments, which however the sceptic may deny them, or the enthusiast disfigure them, are yet, I am convinced, original and component parts of the human soul; those senses of the mind which connect us with, and link us to, those awful obscure realities-and an all-powerful, and equally beneficent God.[36]

In a letter to Mrs Dunlop 31st January 1796 he is again personal:

I have lately drunk deep of the cup of affliction. The autumn robbed me of my only daughter and darling child, and that at a distance too, and so rapidly, as to put it out of my power to pay the last duties to her. I had scarcely begun to recover from that shock, when I became myself the victim of severe rheumatic fever, and long the die spun doubtful; until, after many weeks of a sick bed, it seems to have turned up life, and I am beginning to crawl across the room, and once indeed have been before my own door in the street.[37]

And to Mr Thomson, April 1796:

. . . almost ever since I wrote to you last: I have only known existence by the pressure of the heavy hand of sickness, and have counted time by the repercussions of pain! Rheumatism, cold, and fever have formed to me a terrible combination. I close my eyes in misery, and open them without hope.[38]

In a letter to Mr Thomson, Burns writes (the letter undated) 'I have reason to believe that my complaint is the flying gout.'[39]This probably refers to rheumatic pains moving around the body, sometimes known as flitting pains, the word 'gout' being used in a generic sense.

To Mrs Burns, Brow on the Solway Firth Thursday 1796:

I delayed writing until I could tell what effect sea-bathing was likely to produce. It would be injustice to deny that it has eased my pains, and, I think, has strengthened me; but my appetite is still extremely bad. Nor flesh nor fish can I swallow; porridge and milk are the only things I can taste.[40]

Mrs Dunlop Brow 12th July 1796:

An illness which has long hung about me, in all probability will speedily send me beyond that 'bourn whence no traveller returns'. . . . you conversation, and especially your correspondence, were at once highly entertaining and instructive. With what pleasure did I use to break up the seal! The remembrance yet adds one pulse more to my poor palpitating heart.[41]

Burns died on 21st July 1796.

While these comments do not constitute a formal diary of a dying man they can be compared to other diaries such as *Diary of a Dying Man* by William Soutar, which will be discussed subsequently.[42] They do however give a clear statement of his condition.

Quality of life and happiness

In 'Contented wi' Little and Canty wi' Mair' (1799) Burns sets the scene and the theme which is re-stated on many occasions; that quality of life and happiness are not only, or perhaps at all, associated with wealth, riches, status and power. Life is more than material matters and concerns many more aspects of a persons being:

> Contented wi little, and cantie wi mair,
> Whene'er I forgather wi Sorrow and Care,
> I gie them a skelp, as they're creepin alang,
> Wi a cog o guid swats and an auld Scottish sang.[43]

In 'A Man's a Man for a' That' (1795) he goes even further and in politically loaded terms:

> Is there for honest poverty
> That hings his head, an a' that?
> The coward slave, we pass him by –
> We dare be poor for a' that!
> For a' that, an a' that,
> Our toils obscure, an a'that,
> The rank is but the guinea's stamp,
> The man's the gowd for a' that.

Ye see yon birkie ca'd 'a lord,'
Wha struts, an stares, an a' that?
Tho hundreds worship at his word,
He's but a cuif for a' that.
For a' that, an a' that,
His ribband, star, an a' that,
The man o independent mind,
He looks an laughs at a' that.

Then let us pray that come it may
(As come it will for a' that)
That Sense and Worth o'er a' the earth,
Shall bear the gree an a' that.
For a' that, an a' that,
It's comin yet for a' that,
That man to man, the world, o'er
Shall brithers be for a' that.[44]

Here is an impassioned plea for equity, and an emphasis on honesty, sense, worth, and independence of mind. Hard work has its own rewards, and even if these rewards are meagre they still matter in crystallising quality of life for the individual and the family.

This perspective is even more explicitly set out in the 'Epistle to Davie, a brother poet' (1786):

It's no in titles nor in rank;
It's no in wealth like Lon'on Bank
To purchase peace and rest,
It's no in makin muckle, mair;
It's no in books, it's no in lear,
To make us truly blest:
If happiness hae not her seat
An centre in the breast,
We may be wise, or rich, or great,
But can never be blest!

106

> Nae treasures nor pleasures
> Could make us happy lang;
> The heart's ay's the part ay
> That makes us right or wrang[45]

This is a most powerful statement of the nature of happiness and well-being. Peace and rest don't come from wealth or power, or even learning. They come from deep inside us. Happiness is centred in the heart.

But perhaps most poignantly are the lines in 'To a Mouse' (1786):

> Still thou are blest, compar'd wi me!
> The present only toucheth thee:
> But och! I backward cast my e'e,
> On prospects drear!
> An forward, tho I canna see,
> I guess an fear![46]

It is difficult to predict the future, and our plans sometimes go haywire. But the mouse, now dead, is blessed compared with the ploughman. The troubles of the mouse are over, but the man looks ahead to poor prospects, and while it is not possible to see into the future, it is full of fear. The human mind can imagine the bad things ahead, and can only dread the years ahead.

'The Twa Dogs' (1786) repeats the theme. As the ploughman's dog Luath suggest of humble folk:

> They're no sae wretched's ane wad think:
> Tho' constantly on poortith's brink,
> They're sae accustom'd wi the sight,
> The view o't gies them little fright.
> Then chance and fortune are sae guided,
> They're ay in less or mair provided;
> And tho fatigu'd wi close employment,
> A blink o rest's a sweet enjoyment.
> The dearest comfort o their lives,
> Their gushie weans an faithfu wives;

> The prattling things are just their pride,
> That sweetens a' their fireside.

Here we note the things that bring comfort; children and families, rest by the fireside and good conversation.

In 'Verses in Friars' Carse Heritage' (1788) the narrator picks up the theme of happiness and contemplates that:

> Happiness is but a name,
> Make content and ease thy aim.
> Ambition is a meteor-gleam;
> Fame a restless idle dream;
> Pleasures, insects on the wing
> Peace, th' tend'rest flow'r of spring,
> Those that sip the dew alone –
> Make the butterflies thy own;
> Those that would the bloom devour –
> Crush the locusts, save the flower.[47]

This powerful statement on the issues of ambition and the search for fame contrasts with peace and simple, natural pleasures. He also notes how readily such pleasures can be crushed.

Burns recognises further how evanescent pleasure and happiness can be in 'Tam o'Shanter':

> But pleasures are like poppies spread:
> You seize the flow'r, its bloom is shed;
> Or like the snow falls in the river,
> A moment white – then melts for ever;
> Or like the borealis race,
> That flit ere you can point their place;
> Or like a rainbow's lovely form
> Evanishing amid the storm.
> Nae man can tether time or tide,
> The hour approaches Tam maun ride

Once again the ephemeral nature of pleasure described in several ways. The final two lines noting that one can't just sit and wait for happiness to come, action may be required.

'Auld Lang Syne' (1796) has three relevant verses, not often sung, but poignant reminders of what happiness was, what pleasure we had, and why friends and memories matter:

> We twa hae run about the braes,
> And pou'd the gowans fine,
> But we've wander'd monie a weary fit,
> Sin auld lang syne.
>
> We twa hae paidl'd in the burn
> Frae morning sun till dine,
> But seas between us braid hae roar'd
> Sin auld lang syne.'
>
> And there's a hand my trusty fiere,
> And gie's a hand o thine,
> And we'll tak a right guid-willie waught,
> For auld lang syne.[48]

These lines look back to what mattered most in our lives; family friends, being together. It is almost like going through an old photograph album and smiling at the memories of how things were. Friends are so important and the handshake a sign of such a friendship.

So how would Burns have defined happiness and quality of life? How do his writings help us to improve both? Are there any clues to a positive way forward? It is clear that Burns considers that it is possible to be happy without rank, power, learning or wealth. Ambition can get in the way, as can the search for fame. Accruing possessions and wealth may have negative benefit. A search for pleasure will not satisfy entirely and is evanescent. On the other hand his comments on poverty suggest that at the extreme this too is not conducive to happiness. This chimes with a verse in Alan Ramsay's 'The Gentle Shepherd'[49]

> He that has just enough can soundly sleep;

So what is happiness? Honest toil, friendship, family and a nice warm fire? Is that all it takes to be happy? Burns makes the point that happiness emanates from deep inside and we can never be best unless the heart feels it. Perhaps more forcefully in 'A Man's a Man for a' That' the poet makes the point that it is also about being part of a society that helps each other, and the real objective is to be part of a worldwide brotherhood. This echoes a contemporary, Adam Smith, in the *Theory of Moral Sentiments* (1759):

> How selfish soever man may be supposed, there are evidently some principles in his nature, which interest him in the fortunes of others, though he derives nothing from it but the pleasure of seeing it. [50]

Pertinently this comes from Adam Smith whom Burns read voraciously as he took advantage of the philosophical wisdom of the Scottish Enlightenment.

Learning

In my introduction, I made a case for learning to be at the heart of changing health and quality of life. In this section, I want to demonstrate how Burns sets out his own views on learning, within the context of the Scottish Enlightenment.

Burns recognises Scotland's place in the pursuit of learning. In 'The Prologue spoken by Mr Woods on his benefit night', 16th April 1787' he sets the theme out well:

> But here's an ancient nation, fam'd afar
> For genius, learning high, as great in war.
> Hail, Caledonia! Name for ever dear!
> Before whose sons I'm honor'd to appear!
> Where every science, every nobler art,
> That can inform the mind or mend the heart,
> Is known (a grateful nations oft have found),
> Far as the rude barbarian marks the bound!
> Philosophy, no idle pedant dream,
> Here holds her search by heaven-taught Reason's beam. [51]

A declaration of the learning in Scotland in the 18th century; from philosophy to the sciences, the mend the mind and heart, and to bring reason to decision making.

The poet knew many of the great names of the day as reflected in 'Lament for the absence of William Creech, Publisher: (1787)'. The narrator pines:

> Nae mair we see his levee door
> Philosophers and Poets pour,
> And toothy Critics by the score,
> In bloody raw:
> The adjutant o a' the core,
> Willie's awa!

> Now worthy Greg'ry's Latin face,
> Tytler's and Greenfield's modest grace,
> M'Kenzie, Stewart, such a brace
> As Rome ne'er saw,
> They a' maun meet some ither place —
> Willie's awa!

A list of names mentioned which summarise some of the great intellects of the Enlightenment, and illustrates Burns' familiarity with them.

In 'The Epistle to Robert Graham of Fintry' (1788) he notes again the importance of learning, recognising first the importance of the mind: 'When nature her great master-piece design'd / And framed her last, best work, the human mind.'[52] He then lays out the occupations and skills available:

> The useful many first, she calls them forth -
> Plain, plodding Industry and sober Worth;
> Thence peasants, farmers, native sons of earth,
> And merchandise' whole genus take their birth;
> Each prudent cit a warm existence finds,
> And all mechanics' many-apron'd kinds.
> Some other rarer sorts are wanted yet —
> The lead and buoy are needful to the net:

> The caput mortuum of gross desires
> Makes a material for mere knights and squires;
> The martial phosphorus is taught to flow;
> She kneads the lumpish philosophic dough,
> Then marks th' unyielding mass with grave designs –
> Law, physic, politics, and deep divines;
> Last, she sublimes th' Aurora of the poles,
> The flashing elements of female souls.

He completes the list by ensuring that the poet is the highest form of being, perhaps in jest, though there is a serious point here about the role of the poet in drawing together the strands of life.

There are numerous interesting references in this poem, to law, medicine and divinity, for example. The reference in the text to phosphorus is of particular interest. How could such an 'Unlettered ploughman' know about such an element and its properties? There may be a clue in the letters between Burns and Mrs Dunlop. In her letter to Burns dated the end of August 1788, she notes:

> I begin to fear your fire has gone out, and you were going to light up a new one of turpentine and the marine, and a very unodoriferous flame and dangerous to its neighbours, as I once experienced in attending a course of experiments in Natural Philosophy. The operator told us on mixing the three coldest liquids in the world there would arise a sudden flame . . . Instantly a blaze of liquid fire poring over the table on every side, accompanied by the most suffocating exhalation, made everyone run out of the room as fast as possible. . . . Next day I had the honour to be where Lord Stair was long expected. At length he appeared, and apologised for his absence . . . he had been obliged to wait till my lady had darned holes burnt in them (his clothes) at yesterday's exhibition.[53]

Later in a letter of the 12th September 1788 she refers to the poem itself on which she has been asked to comment by Burns:

> I hope and believe your lines must please the man to whom they are addrest (Epistle to Robert Graham of Fintry) . . . there is a great variety of finely

fancied epithets thrown through the whole . . . and though I would have wished you less hard on the poor knights and squires, I much admire the flowing phosphorus and lumpish dough and unyielding mass, and most of all the flashing borealis[54]

Mrs Dunlop may be referring in her letter of the end of August, to Professor John Anderson (1726–1796), known to his students as 'Jolly Jack Phosphorus', and who was born in Rosneath in Dunbartonshire. He became Professor of Oriental languages at Glasgow University, then in 1757 became Chair of Natural Philosophy. He believed strongly in 'useful learning' for the working classes by providing lectures in the evenings for both men and women. In these he used experiments to demonstrate the power of science, and used to set off explosions and fireworks, hence his nickname. Could this have been the event referred to in Mrs Dunlop's account of the explosions in the presence of Lord Stair? Anderson disliked the university and bequeathed his property to found a school of 'useful Learning' which has subsequently become, over the centuries, the University of Strathclyde.

In the 'Epistle to J. Lapraik' (1786) Burns nails his colours firmly to the mast in terms of motivation to learn:

> What's a' your jargon o your schools,
> Your Latin names for horns an stools?
> If honest Nature made you fools,
> What sairs your grammars?
> Ye'd better taen up spades and shools
> Or knappin-hammers
>
> A set o dull, conceited hashes
> Confuse their brains in college-classes,
> They gang in stirks, and come out asses
> Plain truth to speak;
> An syne they think to climb Parnassus
> By dint o Greek!

> Gie me ae spark o' Nature's fire,
> That's a' the learning I desire;
> Then, tho I drudge thro dub and mire
> At pleugh or cart,
> My Muse, tho hamely in attire,
> May touch the heart.[55]

This is perhaps Burns at his most passionate about learning. All he needs is a 'spark of Nature's fire' to help him write his muse. In clinical terms it is the same. A problem presented and unsolved, symptoms not understood, a chance observation, a curious mind, have all set off voyages of discovery and inventions. Curiosity remains an instinct to be instilled in all those interested in improving health and quality of life. It is reflected in a passion for lifelong learning.

In the 'The Holy Fair' (1786) he takes a more light-hearted look at learning:

> Leeze me on drink! It gies me mair
> Than either school or college;
> It kindles wit, it waukens lear,
> It pangs us fou o knowledge:
> Be't whisky-gill or penny wheep,
> Or onie stronger potion,
> It never fails, on drinkin deep,
> To kittle up our notion,
> By night or day.[56]

Here is a wonderful reference to the supposed learning power of alcohol; it sparks the imagination, helps learning and gives us real insight.

In 'The Ordination' (1787) the poet sees a side of knowledge which may be less useful unless linked to common sense:

> There, Learning, with his Greekish face,
> Grunts out some Latin ditty;
> And Common-sense is gaun she says,

Robert Burns, remember Tam o' Shanter's mare

To mak to Jamie Beattie

Her plaint this day[57]

His views in this extract reflect those in some of his other works; Greek and Latin identified with learning, while common sense, in the shape of the Philosopher James Beattie, is the one to look out for. Knowledge of Greek and Latin may be outward signs of learning and wisdom, what is just as relevant is common sense.

The 'Epistle to James Tennant of Glenconner' (1802) shows Burns' remarkable range of interests and knowledge of Enlightenment Scotland. The narrator says:

> I've sent you here, by Johnie Simson,
> Twa sage philosophers to glimpse on:
> Smith, wi his sympathetic feeling,
> An Reid, to common sense appealing.
> Philosophers have fought and wrangled,
> And meikle Greek an Latin mangled.
> Till, wi their logic-jargon tir'd
> And in the depth of science mir'd,
> To common sense they now appeal –
> What wives and wabsters see and feel![58]

A reference again to common sense and the reflection that the Scottish School of Commonsense Philosophy and the Academy had now caught up with 'wives and wabsters' and that learning had now caught up with the real world.

The reference to Adam Smith is of importance. In Burns' commonplace book written between 1783 and 1785 he notes: 'I entirely agree with that judicious philosopher Mr Smith in his excellent Theory of Moral Sentiments, that remorse is the most painful sentiment that can embitter the human bosom'.[59] This is a personal reflection of some aspects of Burns' life, perhaps related to the things he had, or had not, done

There is one further intriguing aspect of Burns and the academic world, revealed again in the correspondence with Mrs Dunlop – could Burns have become an academic? In a letter dated 1st April 1789, she draws Burns' attention to 'your friend Creech's advertisement in the *Edr. Courant* for proposals about a professor of Agriculture'. Dunlop goes on in the same letter 'I would have you give this a little serious attention, since I do not believe there is a man in the kingdom who might so properly blend the theoretical and practical knowledge that plan would seem to require.'[60]

Not only that, it would also change his status, 'besides Edina would not be so irksome when one was not from home there, nor would a grave member of the College be so oft the prey of jolly Bacchus as an Exciseman, at least against his will.'[61]

Burns replies on the 21st April 1789 'I believe the professorship will be an idle project; but whatever it may be, I, or such as I, am quite out of the question.'[62] Mrs Dunlop replies on the 23rd April, 'I am assured the professorship is unappropriated, even in idea. It is endowed by Mr Poulteney. I wish to God he thought of both you and it as I do, and it would be yours, at least if you wish it to be so; but perhaps you have an aversion to it.'[63]

The chair was to be funded by the Pulteney Family, and in 1790, a year later, the first Professor, Dr Andrew Coventry of Shanwell was appointed. For Burns, this would have been a possible change of profession, and have propelled him into the world of formal learning. It would have been interesting to see how this would have reflected on his poems and songs that would have appeared afterwards.

In some of his writings there are suggestions that not only had he read widely, but was interested in the importance of books and reading as the earlier reference to his letter to Sir John Sinclair shows. In addition he asks for some help in getting copies from Mr Hill, in relation to the Monkland Friendly Society and their library. There are also comments from Burns that the might have aspirations to be a literary critic. For example it has already been mentioned that Burns was given a present of *Zeluco* by John Moore and he notes, 'In fact I have gravely planned a comparative view of you, Fielding, Richardson and Smollett, in your different qualities and merits as novel writers.'[64]

He makes a fascinating reference to Allan Ramsay and the 'Gentle Shepherd' in a letter to Mr Cunningham 1792. 'Bye the Bye, do you know Allan? He must be a man of very great genius-Why is he not more known? Has he no Patrons? Or do 'Poverty's cold wind and crushing wind beat keen and heavy' on him?'[65]This comment again notes his links with the wider community, but also reflects on his concerns for others and the ever present problems of poverty.

Conclusions

Burns in his poems and letters shows remarkable depth and breadth of insight into the human condition and the problems of health and illness in 18th century Scotland. Of particular interest are his views on quality of life and happiness. The debate still rumbles on about such matters and there are questionnaires and surveys which estimate just how happy we are. There is still much to learn from Burns on such matters. The Enlightenment was a special time in Scotland and Burns made full use of the ambience and the connections he made in his poetry. His links with the medical profession were extensive and his comments on them – good and bad – are revealing. He almost became an academic, yet was clearly happiest as a poet, writing about everyday common people and events, endowing and memorialising them with his special language and imagination.

Notes

1   'Tam O'Shanter', in *The Complete PoeticalWorks of Robert Burns,* pp. 410–15, ll. 221–26.

2   Richard Griffin, ed., *The Letters of Robert Burns* (Glasgow: Richard Griffin and Co., 1828); William Wallace, ed., *Robert Burns and Mrs Dunlop: Correspondence now published in full* (London: Hodder and Stoughton, 1898); William Findlay, *Robert Burns and the Medical Profession* (London: Alexander Gardiner, 1898); Robert DonaldThornton, *William Maxwell to Robert Burns* (Edinburgh: John Donald Publishers, 1979).

3   William Buchan, *Buchan's Domestic Medicine, or a Treatise on the Prevention and Cure of Disease by Regimen and Simple Medicines* (Edinburgh: Arch Allardice, 1824).

4   'Death and Doctor Hornbook', in *The Complete Poetical Works of Robert Burns*, pp. 96–100, ll. 79–84.

5   W.F. Bymun and R. Porter, *Companion Encyclopaedia of the History of Medicine* (London and NewYork: Routledge, 1993), II, pp. 1297–9.

6   Buchan, *Domestic Medicine*, p. 477.

7   'The Fete Champetre', in *The Complete PoeticalWorks of Robert Burns,* pp. 326–7, ll. 1–8.

8   'Address to the unco guid, or the rigidly righteous', in *The Complete Poetical Works of Robert Burns*, pp. 74–76, ll. 33–40.

9   Office for National Statistics. *Lifestyle Survey Overview. A Report of the 2010 General Lifestyle Survey* (Newport: National Statistics Publication, 2012).

10   'To a Louse', in *The Complete Poetical Works of Robert Burns*, pp. 181–2, ll. 37–42.

11   'Tam O'Shanter', in *The Complete Poetical Works of Robert Burns*, pp. 410–15, ll. 221–26.

12   'Letter of Robert Burns to Mrs Dunlop, 25 January 1790', in Wallace, *Robert Burns and Mrs Dunlop*, p. 237.

13   Ibid., '17 February 1791', p. 303.

14   Ibid., '17 February 1791', p. 314.

15   'Letter of John Hunter to Edward Jenner, 2 August 1775', in Hunter, John, *Works of John Hunter*, 4 vols (London: Longman, Rees, Orme, Brown, Green and Longman, 1835–1837), I, p. 65.

16   'Letter of Robert Burns to Sir John Sinclair', undated, in Griffin, *The Letters of Robert Burns*, p.145–7.

17   'Scotch Drink', in *The Complete Poetical Works of Robert Burns*, pp. 165–8.

18   'The Twa Dogs', in *The Complete Poetical Works of Robert Burns*, pp. 140–6.

19   'The Cotter's Saturday Night', in *The Complete Poetical Works of Robert Burns*, pp. 147–151.

20   'Address to a Haggis', in *The Complete Poetical Works of Robert Burns*, pp. 264–5, ll. 1–12.

21   'The Shepherd's Wife', in *The Complete Poetical Works of Robert Burns*, pp. 453–4.

22   Findlay, *Robert Burns and the Medical Profession*.

23   'A Dream', in *The Complete Poetical Works of Robert Burns*, p. 233–4, ll. 30–31.

24   'To Robert Graham of Fintry', in *The Complete Poetical Works of Robert Burns*, pp. 431–2, ll. 37–40.

25   William Shakespeare, *Romeo and Juliet*, V.1, in *William Shakespeare: The Collected Works*, eds. Stanley Wells, Gary Taylor, John Jowett and William Montgomery (Oxford: Clarendon Press, 1988).

26   'Epistle to John Goldie, in Kilmarnock', in *The Complete Poetical Works of Robert Burns*, pp. 121–2, ll. 7–18.

27   'Letter of Robert Burns to Mr Thomson, September 1974', Griffin, *The Letters of Robert Burns*, pp. 283–4.

28   'Letter of Robert Burns to William Creech, 30 May 1789', in Griffin, *The Letters of Robert Burns*, p. 346.

29   'Address to the Toothache', in *The Complete Poetical Works of Robert Burns*, pp. 553, ll. 1–30.

30   Buchan, *Domestic Medicine*, pp. 115–122. See also: T.Chin and P.D. Welsby, 'Malaria

in the UK: Past, Present and future', *Postgraduate Medical Journal*, 80 (2004), 663–6; J.H. Bayliss, 'Epidemiological Considerations of the History of Indigenous Malaria in Britain', *Endeavour*, 9 (1985), 191–4; K. Duncan and Proc.R. Coll, 'The Possible Influence of Climate Change on Historical Outbreaks of Malaria in Scotland', *Physicians Edinb.*, 23 (1993), 55–62; J. Roy, 'Malaria in England Past, Present and Future', *Soc Promotion of Health*, 94 (1974), 23–9.

31 'Libel Summons', in *The Complete Poetical Works of Robert Burns*, pp. 227–230, ll. 61–82.

32 'John Anderson, My Jo', in *The Complete Poetical Works of Robert Burns*, p. 391.

33 'What can a young lassie do wi' an auld man', in *The Complete Poetical Works of Robert Burns*, pp. 441–2, ll. 5–8.

34 'Man was Made to Mourn', in *The Complete Poetical Works of Robert Burns*, pp. 123–5, ll. 57–64.

35 'Tam Samson's Elegy', in *The Complete Poetical Works of Robert Burns*, pp. 239–241, ll. 49–64.

36 *The letters of Robert Burns* pp. 273–4.

37 Ibid, 'Letter of Robert Burns to Mrs Dunlop, 31 January 1796', p. 311.

38 Ibid, 'Letter of Robert Burns to Mr Thomson, April 1796', p. 314.

39 Ibid. 'Letter of Robert Burns to Mr Thomson', undated, p. 314.

40 Ibid, 'Letter of Mrs Burns to Robert Burns, Thursday 1796', p. 317.

41 Ibid, 'Letter of Robert Burns to Mrs Dunlop, 12 July 1796', p. 318.

42 William Soutar, *Diaries of a Dying Man*, ed. Alexander Scott (Edinburgh: W & R Chambers, 1954).

43 'Contented wi' little and canty wi' mair', in *The Complete Poetical Works of Robert Burns*, pp. 531–2, ll. 1–4.

44 Ibid, 'A man's a man for a'that', pp. 535–36, ll. 1–40.

45 Ibid, 'Epistle to Davie, a brother poet', pp. 86–9, ll. 57–70.

46 Ibid, 'To a mouse', pp. 131–2, ll. 37–48.

47 Ibid, 'Verses in friars' carse hermitage', p. 324, ll. 9–18.

48 Ibid, 'Auld Lang Syne', p. 431, ll. 13–24.

49 Alan Ramsay, *The Gentle Shepherd*, (Edinburgh: George Reid, Printers, 1798), p16.

50 Adam Smith, *The Theory of Moral Sentiments*, ed. D.D. Raphael and A.L. Macfie (Indianapolis: Liberty Fund, 1984), p. 9.

51 'The Prologue spoken by Mr Woods on his benefit night', in *The Complete Poetical Works of Robert Burns,* pp. 275–6, ll. 9–18.

52 Ibid, 'The Epistle to Robert Graham', pp. 330–3, ll. 1–2.

53 'Letter of Mrs Dunlop to Robert Burns, August 1788', Griffin, *Robert Burns and Mrs Dunlop*, p. 89.

54 Ibid, 'Letter of Mrs Dunlop to Robert Burns, 12 September 1788', p. 93.

55 'Epistle to J. Lapraik', in *The Complete Poetical Works of Robert Burns,* pp. 101–4, ll. 55–72.

56 Ibid, 'The Holy Fair', pp. 135–9, ll. 163–171.

57 Ibid, 'The Ordination', pp. 192–4, ll. 95–9.

58 Ibid, 'Epistle to James Tennant of Glenconner' pp. 200–202, ll. 7–16.

59 Burns, *Commonplace Book*, p. 7.

60 'Letter of Mrs Dunlop, 1 April 1989', in Wallace, *Robert Burns and Mrs Dunlop*, p. 160.

61 Ibid.

62 Ibid, p. 166.

63 Ibid, p. 167.

64 'Letter of Robert Burns to John Moore, 14 July 1790', Griffin, *The Letters of Robert Burns*, p. 163.

65 Ibid, 'Letter of Robert Burns to Mr Cunningham, 2 March 1792', p. 200.

CHAPTER 9

Tobias Smollett (1721–1771)

Pills are good for nothing – I might as well swallow snowballs to cool my veins

The Expedition of Humphrey Clinker

Introduction

Tobias Smollett was born in 1721 in Renton, Dunbartonshire. He was educated at the University of Glasgow and trained as a surgeon in that city. He moved to London where he tried to establish himself as a writer, then he became a ship's surgeon in the Royal Navy, travelling to Jamaica where he settled down for a few years. On returning the London he set up practice in Downing Street and married a wealthy Jamaican heiress, Anna Lascelles. He died in 1771 and there is a memorial to him in Renton in front of Renton Primary School. The Latin inscription notes that he is interred far away in Leghorn in Italy, but the monument is erected where he was born. The memorial was not given for him alone, but to encourage others. The text of the inscription is discussed in the *Journal of a Tour to the Hebrides* by James Boswell in the entry for the 28th October 1773, and Dr Johnson was consulted on whether there should be a Latin translation, to which Johnson replied, 'no'.

His most popular works were *The Adventures of Roderick Random* (1748), *The Expedition of Humphry Clinker* (1771) and *The Adventures of Peregrine Pickle* (1751), and two of these will be discussed here, but there were many other literary productions.

While Smollett was in Glasgow he made important links and some have been referred to in the chapter on Robert Burns. One of the most significant was Dr John Moore (his son, Sir John Moore of Corunna, born on Donald's Land, became a hero during the Napoleonic wars). Dr Moore was a friend of Tobias Smollett, who was a little older than he was, and who was learning his medical trade in Dr Gordon's surgery in Gibson's Land at the corner of Saltmarket and Prince's Street, where Moore had also been an apprentice.

Smollett's *Humphry Clinker* may have been written over a period of four years with some evidence that he may have made notes on it in Scotstoun House in Glasgow, and that one of the rooms was called 'Smollett's Study'.[1] The house is now long gone, though there is an interesting link with Burns. In 1789 Burns was going to Ayrshire and put up at the inn for the night in Sanquhar, when the funeral cortege of Mrs Oswald of Auchincruive came past. He was forced to leave the inn and drive on, and he wrote a few uncomplimentary verses to Mrs Oswald who had owned the House at Scotstoun.

Smollett was in touch with many doctors in the 18th century but there is one special note from Smollett to Dr John Hunter, written in 1771, which is worth noting. Smollett writes:

> With respect to myself, I have nothing to say, but that if I can prevail upon my wife to execute my last will, you shall receive my poor carcase in a box, after I am dead, to be placed among your rarities. I am already so dry and emaciated, that I may pass for an Egyptian mummy without any other dry preparation than some pitch and painted linen, unless you think I may deserve the denomination of a curiosity in my own character.[2]

I have pursued this note both in London and Glasgow but no evidence has been found in either Hunterian Museum that his body was left for study.

The Expedition of Humphry Clinker

This story, written as an epistolary novel, records the travels of a family group around Britain. It notes their habits, their food, their illnesses and the character of the places and people. Because of Smollett's medical education there are numerous detailed references to medical issues, including diseases and their treatment. It is a remarkable resource of medical practice and of the determinants of health in the 18th century.

In the first letter in the book Bramble (the central character) writes to his doctor complaining and sets the scene for subsequent correspondence:

> The pills are good for nothing – I might as might as well swallow snowballs to cool my veins – I have told you over and over, how hard I am to move; and at this time of the day, I ought to know something of my own constitution. Why will you be so positive? Prithee send me another prescription.

The travellers are always looking for new insights into medical practice and Smollett uses some very vivid examples. These include the importance of 'temperament' in the novel. For example, J. Melford writes to Sir Watkin Phillips:

> The learned Dr B– (Dr Edward Barry) in his treatise on the Four Digestions, explains in what manner the volatile effluvia from the intestines, stimulate and promote the operations of the animal oeconomy: he affirmed, the last Grand Duke of Tuscany, of the Medicis family . . . was so delighted with that odour, that he caused the essence of that ordure to be extracted, and used it as the most delicious perfume: that he himself (the doctor) when he happened to be low spirited, or fatigued with business, found immediate relief and uncommon satisfaction from hanging over the stale contents of a close-stool while his servants stirred it under his nose.

This is an early example of aromatherapy, a range of treatments used in clinical pratice, though this one may not be used frequently.

Another strange example is when they are at the Hot Baths in Bath, and the patient is confirmed as having a 'dropsical habit' (abdominal fluid). It may need to be tapped to remove it and the comment, by the same J. Melford, is:

> If I should be present when it is tapped, I will give convincing proof of what I assert, by drinking without hesitation the water that comes out of your abdomen. The ladies made wry faces at this declaration.

This comment is made without any real physiological basis, except that in heart failure such fluid accumulation in the abdomen is made worse by drinking.

The impotence of the doctor and the lack of understanding at the time of science and disease are well illustrated by another letter to Dr Lewis, Bramble writes:

> There are mysteries in physick, as well as in religion; which we of the profane have no right to investigate. A man must not presume to use his reason, unless he has studied the categories, and can chop logic by mode and figure . . . For my own part I have had a hospital these fourteen years within myself, and studied my own case with the most painful attention; consequently I may be supposed to know something of the mater, although I have not taken regular courses of physiology etc. I short, I have for sometime been of the opinion, (no offence dear Doctor) that the sum of all your medical discoveries amounts to this, that the more you study the less you know.

The hygiene in the baths also comes under scrutiny. Bramble goes to the baths to cleanse his skin, and again writes to Dr Lewis, with an interesting use of the term virus:

> The first object that saluted my eye, was a child full of scrophulous ulcers (probably tuberculosis), carried in the arms of one of the guides, under the very noses of the bathers. I was so shocked at the sight, that I retired immediately with indignation and disgust – suppose the matter of those ulcers, floating on the water, comes into contact with my skin, when the pores are all open? I would ask what must be the consequences? . . . we must all imbibe the king's evil, the scurvy, the cancer and the pox. . . . no doubt, the heat will render the virus the more volatile and penetrating.

There are many more examples of the conditions which prevailed and one interesting comment on the individuals who frequented the baths. When he goes to the coffee house one afternoon Bramble can not help contemplating the company. As he writes again to Dr Lewis,

> We consisted of thirteen individuals; seven lamed by gout, rheumatism

or palsy, three maimed by accident; and the rest either deaf or blind. One hobbled another hopped, a third dragged his legs after him like a wounded snake, a fourth straddled betwixt a long pair of crutches.

The very modern description of this group of older travellers is one which might still be replicated today.

There is also a key reference to the British Museum and the creation of the collection which becomes the British Library:

It would likewise be a great improvement, with respect to the library, if the deficiencies were made up, by purchasing all the books of character that are not already found in the collection – they might be classed in centuries, according to the dates of their publication, and catalogues printed of them and the manuscripts, for the information of those that want to consult or compile from such authorities. I could also wish, for the honour of the nation, that there was a complete apparatus for a course of mathematics, mechanics, and experimental philosophy; and a good salary settled upon and able professor, who should give regular lectures on these subjects.

This early description of the making of a library and the uses to which it might be harnessed is impressive. In particular the educational and learning functions are emphasised.

There is also a clear comment on environmental issues of the day. Bramble lives in the country with clean air and water, sleeps well in the quiet, listening only to the birds. He eats fresh food and vegetables. Nor does he take less pleasure in seeing his tenants thriving under his auspices. The poor live comfortably under his care, and they have employment. He contrasts this with London:

I am pent up in frowzy lodgings, where there is not enough room to swing a cat; and I breathe the streams of endless putrefaction: and these would, undoubtedly, produce a pestilence, if they were not qualified by the gross acid of sea-coal, which is itself a pernicious nuisance to lungs of any delicacy of texture . . . I go to bed after midnight, jaded and restless from the dissipations of the day – I start every hour from my sleep, at the horrid noise of the watchmen bawling the hour through every street, and thundering at every door. . . . If I would drink water I must quaff the maukish contents of an open aqueduct, exposed to all manner of defilement; or swallow that which comes from the river Thames, impregnated with all the filth of London and Westminster-human excrement is the least offensive part of the concrete, which is composed of all the drugs, minerals and poisons used by mechanics and manufacture, enriched by the putrefying carcasses of men and beasts.

He then describes the meat, fish and fruit available. Even the beer would make you vomit.

There are interesting references to hospital development and to Guy's hospital in particular. He notes that there are in London a number of destitute authors and makes the comment that:

I think Guy, who was himself a bookseller, ought to have appropriated one wing or ward of his hospital to the use of decayed authors; though indeed, there is neither hospital, college nor workhouse, within the bills of mortality, large enough to contain the poor of this society, composed, as it is, from the refuse of every other profession.

When the party arrive in Harrogate they meet a lawyer who is an invalid. But it is observed that he ate well and that 'though his bottle was marked *stomachic tincture* he had recourse to it so often, and seemed to swallow it with such relish, that I suspected that it was not compounded in the apothecary's shop, or in the chemist's laboratory.'

So one day, while the lawyer was busy, the labels had been exchanged, and his tasted like an excellent claret. The lawyer at last took the exchanged bottle, tasted it and was found out. At least he had the wit to record the practical joke played on him by his fellow guests.

With such an experience of baths and spas it is interesting to note the comments from one traveller on the benefits of sea-bathing, an issue of some importance at the time:

You and I have plunged together into the Isis; but the sea is a more noble bath, for health as well as pleasure. You cannot conceive what a flow of spirits it gives, and how it braces every sinew of the human frame. Were I to enumerate half of the diseases which are every day cured by sea-bathing, you might justly say you had received a treatise rather than a letter.

As the touring party travel north there are numerous references to diet and the comment that 'that there was nothing to eat in Scotland but oatmeal and sheep's-heads' is similar to that of the more famous Dr Johnson. Other comments on food are a little more complimentary. For example,

I must own some of their dishes are savoury, and even delicate; but I am not yet Scotchman enough to relish their singed sheep's head and haggice. . . . the last, being a mess of minced lights, livers, suet, oatmeal, onions and pepper, inclosed in a sheep's stomach, had a very sudden effect on mine, and the delicate Mrs Tabby changed colour.

They eat oatcakes and wheaten bread and 'I used to vex poor Murray at Balliol College, by asking if there was really no fruit but turnips in Scotland.'

When they reach Edinburgh they stay in the High Street, 'up four pairs of stairs, the fourth being, in this city, reckoned more genteel than the first. The air is in all probability, the better.' Later, there is reference to discharging effluent from the windows into the streets to the sound of *gardy loo*, and horror at the height of the houses and narrowness of the stairs and the problems of fire and accidents.

He describes the playing of golf with leather balls on the links at Leith. They are filled with feathers and 'struck with such force and dexterity from one hole to another, that they will fly an incredible distance. Of this diversion Scots are so fond, that when the weather permits, you will see a multitude of all ranks, from the senator of justice to the lowest tradesmen, mingled together in their shirts, and following the balls with the utmost eagerness.' Such quotations illustrate the range and depth of city life in Scotland's capital; the food eaten and the state of housing and disposal of refuse. The egalitarian nature of golf is also worth noting, one of the few pastimes in which the different classes participated on the same terms.

He is fulsome in his praise of the University of Edinburgh, especially in the Sciences, the Medical School and the Infirmary,

. . .famous all over Europe – the students of this art have the best opportunity of learning it to perfection, in all its branches, as there are different courses for the theory of medicine, and the practice of medicine; for anatomy, chemistry, botany and the materia medica. . . .What renders this part of the education still more complete, is the advantage of attending the infirmary, which is the best instituted charitable foundation that I ever knew.

There are also poor houses and workhouses and there is not a beggar to be seen within the city. Glasgow had set that example thirty years ago. In addition he meets most of those involved in the Enlightenment in Edinburgh. There is even an opportunity to consult the famous Dr Gregory, a name which crops up in many literary works. Tabitha Bramble (the sister of Matt) is unwell and Dr Gregory recommends the Highland air and the use of goat-milk whey.

While in the north he even manages to meet Mr. Smollett, one of the judges of the commissary court, who lives in a house on the banks of Loch Lomond, fourteen miles from Glasgow. When they reach that city they have the good fortune to be received by Mr Moore, an eminent surgeon, and who is described as 'a facetious companion, sensible and shrewd and with a considerable fund of humour.' Glasgow is described as the pride of Scotland with a university with 'professors in all the different branches of science, liberally endowed and judiciously chosen . . . their mode of education is certainly preferable to ours in some respects – the students are not left to the private instructions of tutors; but taught in public schools or classes, each science by its particular professor or regent.'

Melford also notes the manufacturing going on, not just in Glasgow but all around in Hamilton, Paisley, Renfrew and every other place within a dozen miles.

Smallpox is mentioned in their travel into the Highlands, and here is a reference he to the value of whisky. 'They are used to it from the cradle, and find it an excellent preservative against the winter cold . . . I am told that it is given with great success to infants as a cordial in the confluent smallpox when the eruption seems to flag and the symptoms grow unfavourable.' Other delights in the Highlands include sleeping on heather beds and Melford notes 'indeed I have never slept so much to my satisfaction. I was not only soft and elastic, but the plant, being in flower, diffused an agreeable fragrance, which is wonderfully refreshing and restorative.'

Breakfast sounds overwhelming and includes:

One kit of boiled eggs, a second, full of butter, a third full of cream, an entire cheese made of goat's milk, and earthen pot full of honey; the best part of a ham; a cold venison pasty, a bushel of oatmeal, made in thin cakes and bannocks, with a small wheaten loaf in the middle for the strangers, a large stone bottle full of whisky, another of brandy and a kilderkin of ale. . . . finally a large roll of tobacco was presented by way of desert.

And on returning to the Firth of Clyde they visit Smollett, and Bramble again describes the food:

Do you know how we fare on this Scottish paradise? We make free with our landlords mutton, which is excellent, his poultry yard, his garden, his dairy and his cellar. We have delicious salmon, pike, trout and perch at the door for the taking. The firth of Clyde, on the other side of the hill supplies us with mullet, red and grey, cod, mackarel, whiting, and a variety of sea fish including the finest herring I have ever tasted. We have sweet and juicy beef, and tolerable veal, with delicate bread from the little town of Dunbritton; and plenty of partridge, growse, heath cock and other game in presents.

There are general comments on the Scots as being well fed and clothed, though they dwell in poor huts built of loose stone and turfs, without mortar with a fire place in the middle generally made of an old mill stone and a hole at the top to let the smoke out.

These letters provide a remarkable glimpse of Great Britain in the 18th century, the habits, food, illness clothing, housing and environment. They include the medical remedies of the day, and their ineffectiveness. All of the determinants of health are described, and remain today. The only difference is in the medical advances and in the establishment of a national health service.

Roderick Random

This is the tale of a young man who begins his career in Glasgow as a surgical apprentice and who finds adventure in everything that he does. The story begins as he is offered a university education to study medicine by his uncle, Tom Bowling. He first describes his schooling and his proficiency in Latin and arithmetic, and becomes an excellent scholar. After a series of family squabbles, his uncle takes him in hand:

> Mr Bowling . . . this generous tar determined (though he could ill afford it) to give me university education; and accordingly settled my board and other expenses at a town not many miles distant, famous for its colleges, whither we repaired in a short time.[3]

Following this he becomes a surgical apprentice to Mr Crab in Glasgow whom he first meets in a public house where the surgeon was drinking heavily. During his interview for the post he confesses that he understands a little pharmacy, nor was he ignorant of surgery, which he has studied with 'great pleasure and application'. Crab's response is contemptuous. 'Studied surgery! What? In books I suppose . . . you are too learned for me. . . . can you bleed and give a clyster, spread a plaister and prepare a potion?' Roderick replies in the affirmative and that night is admitted to his house.

The first event recorded in the Crab household is that of a young woman made pregnant by Crab, but who was not happy and persuaded the girl that she was not pregnant, 'but only afflicted with a disorder incident to young women, which he could easily remove.' He gives her medicines to produce an abortion, but these fail. Crab then tells Random that it is time he left to make his fortune in the world, and to leave quickly, and in this way Random is blamed for the pregnancy.

So Random goes to London carrying with him 'One suit of cloaths, half a dozen ruffled shirts, . . . a pocket case of instruments, a small edition of Horace, and Wiseman's Surgery (Richard Wiseman 1622–1676) the foremost surgeon of the period, and Serjeant Chirurgeon to King Charles II, and ten guineas in cash.' He carries with him letters of introduction, including one to his Member of Parliament for his own town. His adventure then begins.

Tobias Smollett (1721–1771)

Random arrives in London wishing to join the navy as a surgeon. He finds that he must pass the exam in the College of Surgeons, and to pay money for the privilege. He eventually reaches Surgeons Hall and registers for the examination. Two weeks later he is at the Hall where he mingles with the crowd waiting outside, when a young man appears looking pale and quivering. He describes to the gathering the questions with the answers he has given. Random is called and taken into a large hall where he sees a dozen grim faces sitting round the table, this scene being the subject of contemporary caricature. The first question he is asked is, 'Where were you born?' When he answers 'Scotland' the reply is 'we have scarce any other countrymen to examine you here. You Scotchmen have overspread us of late as the locusts did Egypt.' He is asked about how long he has trained and when he says he has been an apprentice for three years, the examiner falls into a violent passion and swears it is a shame and a scandal to send such raw boys into the world as surgeons. He is then asked about trepanning a skull and his answers seem to satisfy. The next examiner is more aggressive. He is asked about amputations, and about what would he do at sea if someone had their head shot off! He replies that 'such a case has never come under my observation neither do I remember to have seen any method of cure proposed for such an accident, in any of the systems of surgery I have perused.' Several other questions follow by which time the examiners are arguing with each other until the chairman commands silence and Roderick is ordered to withdraw. He passes but only after he has paid his fee and waited until his change was given. What else would you expect from a Scotchman?

Over the years the form and conduct of the surgical fellowship have changed, though it still remains a formidable hurdle to be overcome. The comment on the number of Scots in London is also an interesting one. All of the university medical schools in Scotland produced graduates whereas in England only Oxford and Cambridge produced a smaller number of graduates. To practice London as a physician as part of the Royal College of Physicians also required that the doctor subscribed to the Anglican confession which meant that Scottish doctors (those who were not Anglicans) therefore could not practice.

Richard Wiseman is the author of *Eight Chirurgical Treatises* and it is a fascinating book.[4] First published on 24th May 1676 the eight books are on Tumours, Ulcers, Diseases of the anus, the Kings Evil, Wounds, Gun shot

131

wounds, Fractures and luxations and the Lues Venera. The most character-istic aspect of the book is the methodological approach; differences, causes, signs, prognostics and cure; systematic way of considering illness. In addi-tion the book is full of 'Observations' separately listed in the index. These are case studies, dealt with by Wiseman and show his skill and highlight the methodological approach, they are fascinating.

Random's encounter with an apothecary (another important profession) is a relevant one. The apothecary notes that his experience of medicine was not great but he was the most expert man in making up medicines. The apothecary's list of medicines is fascinating, all of which he could produce from different ingredients; oil of sweet almonds, balsamic syrup, aqua cin-namomi, etc., and which he could make from much cheaper materials. Thus he could make aqua cinnamomi from Thames water. He could disguise the taste of drugs and he had a secret remedy for venereal disease.

Random eventually joins a ship as a junior surgeon and describes his experiences in a most vivid way:

> Morgan (the surgeon) visited the sick at seven o'clock in the evening, and having ordered what was proper, he assisted in making up prescriptions. When he followed with the medicines into the sick berth or the hospital, and observed the situation of the patients, 'I was much less surprised to find people died on board, than astonished that any of them recovered.'

Here he saw about fifty miserable distempered wretches, suspended in rows, so huddled one on another, that not more than fourteen inches was allotted for each with his bed and bedding. He describes the scene:

> They were deprived of the light of the day as well as fresh air; breathing nothing but a noisome atmosphere of the morbid streams exhaling from their own excrements and diseased bodies, devoured with vermin hatched in the filth that surrounded them, and destitute of every convenience neces-sary for people in that helpless condition.

One case is of special interest in that it sets the scene for more recent ethical discussions. One of the crew, Jack Ratlin, suffers a broken leg, a compound fracture with the bone sticking out. Opinion is divided as to what to do, amputate or try to save it. The debate goes on and the patient clearly wants the limb saved. Random decides he can save it. The patent is overjoyed and confirms that nobody else should touch him. If he dies, his blood should be on his own head. This represents a good example of informed consent. They then saw off the splinter sticking through the skin, reduce the fracture, bind up the wound, apply an eighteen-tailed bandage, and put the leg in a box – *secudundum artem* (according to the rules of the art). Everything goes well, the limb is saved and the cure completed in six weeks.

Numerous other instances are given of the impotence of the doctor and on one occasion the doctor is the butt of wit of others as he tries to explain disease and the various treatments available at the time. Random has a guest with him on one occasion, a Dr Wagtail, and the company soon begin to ask him questions on hoarseness, lowness of spirits and indigestion. Wagtail's response is to explain everything in a very prolix manner and harangue on prognostics, diagnostics, symptomatics, therapeutics, initiation and reple-tion. This sets the company off even more and disorder ensues. Overall, Roderick Random is a marvellous expose of the work of the doctor, his deficiencies, the nature of professional education and practice in the 18th century, all delivered with humour and insight.

Conclusions

This is a remarkable set of observations from someone with a medical background, considering the ills and diseases of the community of the time. It is done with humour and with accurate recording of the events and the responses to the various situations medical people of the time find themselves in. There is much for contemporary medicine to consider in these observations, from the role of the doctor, the competencies required, and the responses of the patients and friends and relatives. The educational requirements have changed over the centuries, and the knowledge base has grown, but the same concerns are there when sitting clinical examinations, and in dealing with seriously ill patients. Smollett's experience as a practi-cal surgeon shows thoughout the text with real examples and remedies. Smollett also has the ability to laugh at himself and other doctors and in doing so he removes some of the mystique of the physician or surgeon. All doctors are still human beings with failings and weaknesses. The novel also demonstrates ill health as a direct result of living conditions and there are occasions where this is still the case today.

Notes

1   Tobias Smollett, Introduction to *The Expedition of Humphry Clinker* (Oxford: Oxford University Press, 1998), p. viii.

2   Ibid, p. ix.

3   Tobias Smollett, *The Adventures of Roderick Random*, ed. Paul-Gabriel Bouce (Oxford: Oxford University Press, 1999), p. 15.

4   Richard Wiseman, *Severall Chirurgical Treatises* (London: [n. pub.], 1676). Later editions are entitled *Eight Chirurgicall Treatises*.

CHAPTER 10

Dr John Armstrong

On exercise

Begin with gentle toils; and, as your nerves
Grow firm, to hardier by just steps aspire.
The prudent, even in every modest walk
At first but saunter; and by slow degrees
Increase their pace.

Dr Armstrong (1709–1779) was born in the Parish of Castleton in Roxburghshire. His father and brother were ministers and his name has strong connections with the history and legends of the Borders. He graduated in Medicine in Edinburgh in 1732 under Monro Primus, the Professor of Anatomy (referred to by Burns as one of the 'Bloody Monroes'). It was in Edinburgh that he began to compose verse, and he moved to London where he worked in a variety of clinical posts, in England and abroad. He was well connected with London writers such as James Thomson and David Mallet. He wrote a number of medical texts, including a parody on medical education entitled *An essay for abridging the study of physick*. However the main work which gained him his literary reputation was a long poem on *The Art of Preserving Health* (1744).[1] A recent critical work on this poem has been published by Adam Budd and it provides an informative background to its context and to related texts.[2]

This long poem has four books covering the health implications of air, diet, exercise and the passions. It is noted that he also made some contribution to Thomson's 'The Castle of Indolence' (1748) where he discusses the problems of sloth.

The poem is dedicated to Hygeia, the goddess of health and this is alluded to in the first stanza:

Daughter of Paeon, queen of every joy
Hygeia; whose indulgent smile sustains,
The various race luxuriant Nature pours,
And on thee immortal essences bestows
Immortal youth: auspicious, O descend.

And later, the charge is to Hygeia,

Without thy cheerful active energy
No rapture swells the breast, no poet sings
No more the maids of Helicon delight
Come with me then, O Goddess heavenly gay!
Begin the song; and let it sweetly flow
And let it wisely teach thy wholesome laws:
How best the fickle fabric to support
Of mortal man; in healthy body how
A healthful mind the longest to maintain

The objectives are clear, the maintainence of a healthy body and mind and to identify what are the conditions and determinants of health.

Book I: On Air

The first topic is that of the quality of the air and the benefits of a clean environment. The scene is set at the beginning of the book:

Ye who amid this feverish world would wear
A body free of pain, of cares of mind
Fly the rank city, shun its turbid air;
Breathe not the chaos of eternal smoke
And volatile corruption, from the dead,
The dying, the sickening, and the living world
Exhal'd, to sully Heaven's transparent dome
With dim mortality. It is not air
That from a thousand lungs reeks back to thine,

Sated with exhalations rank and fell
The spoil of dunghills, and the putrid thaw
Of nature; when from shape and texture
She relapses into fighting elements:
It is not Air, but floats a nauseous mass
    Of all obscene, corrupt offensive things.

The case is then made that polluted air is bad for you, and smells. Armstrong later poses the question 'Did not the acid vigour of the mine, rolled from a thousand chimneys, tame the putrid steams that overswarm the sky. This caustic venom would perhaps corrode those tender cells that draw the vital air. . . or by the drunken venous tubes, that yawns in countless pores o'er all the skin . . . and rouse the heart to every fever's rage.' This reference to smoke is significant as coal mines and the burning of coal, was a phenomenon just beginning in the 18th century. As will be noted in discussions on 19th century Scottish literature, this aspect of health is not well covered in that century, even though the industrial grime was much greater. So what then is the answer? Armstrong suggests visiting or living in the countryside:

While yet you breathe, away; the rural wilds
Invite; the mountains call you, and the vales;
The woods, the streams, and each ambrosial breeze
That fans the ever undulating sky

But what if you need to work or live in the city? Armstrong makes some suggestions:

Umbrageous Ham! But if the busy town
Attract thee still to toil for power or gold,
Sweetly thou mays't thy vacant hours possess
In Hampstead, courted by the western wind
Or Greenwich, wavering o'er the winding flood;
Or lose the world amid the sylvan wilds
Of Dulwich, yet by barbarous arts unspoiled.

Or you could move to the Kentish Hills, or to Essex. However, there is a warning. Don't rest too long if the climate is damp, or there are fogs, as 'Quartana there presides', a reference to malaria in the 'slothful Naiad of the Fens.' This is a reference to Naiad, a nymph who looks over fountains and streams. The symptoms of malaria are then described:

> From such a mixture sprung, this fitful pest
> With feverish blasts subdues the sickening land:
> Cold tremors come, with mighty love of rest,
> Convulsive yawnings, lassitude and pains
> That sting the burden'd brows fatigue the loins
> And rack the joints, and every torpid limb

And the damp air doesn't help:

> . . .the spungy air
> For ever weeps; or, turgid with the weight
> Of water, pours a sounding deluge down.
> Skies such as these let ev'ry mortal shun
> Who dreads the dropsy, palsy, or the gout
> Tertian, corrosive scurvy, or moist catarrh;
> Or any other injury that grows
> From raw spun fibres idle and unstrung.

Malaria is well recorded in England in the 18th century, especially in southern counties. It is often referred to as ague, and as a disease it was noted as endemic until the end of the first world war.[3] Cinchona bark was the only treatment and had been used from the 17th century. In the 1820s the active ingredient, quinine was isolated.

As well as being damp, the air may be too dry, and that alone can have health consequences. It can make you drowsy and make the blood thick and 'unfit to lead its pitchy current thro' the secret mazy channels of the brain. The melancholic fiend (that worst despair of physic) hence the rust complexioned man pursues, the whole blood is dry . . .'

Armstrong shows considerable knowledge of the circulation of the blood, the current diseases prevalent in 18ᵗʰ century London, and the difficulties in managing them. And if all this depresses you he has an easy remedy:

> Meantime at home, with cheerful fires dispel
> The humid air: and let your table smoke
> With solid roast or bak'd; or what the herds
> Of tamer breeds supply; or what the wilds
> Yield to the toilsom pleasures of the chase.
> Generous your wine, the boast of rip'ning years,
> But frugal be your cups; the languid frame
> Vapid and sunk from yesterday's debauch,
> Shrinks from the cold embrace of watry heavens.
> But neither these, nor all Apollo's arts,
> Disarm the dangers of the dropping sky
> Unless with exercise and manly toil
> You brace your nerves and spur the lagging blood.

Eat well, drink a little, relax, but take some exercise. There is advice for house building, to steer clear of fogs, lake or fenland, and to think of being in a sunny situation, open to the south, perhaps on a hill. What a review of the impact of air quality on health, and just as relevant today.

Book II: On Diet

The second book relates to diet, and begins with a clear rationale for the need for food to repair and strengthen the body. He begins again with the physiology of diet and the role of the blood in rejuvenating those parts which have become damaged:

> The blood, the fountain whence the spirits flow
> The generous stream that waters every part,
> And motion, vigour, and warm life conveys
> To every particle that moves or lives;
> This vital fluid, thro' unnumbered tubes
> Pour'd by the heart, and to the heart again
> Refunded; scourged for ever round and round;

139

But the force also repairs and restores and

> For this the watchful appetite was give'n,
> Daily with fresh materials to repair
> This unavoidable expense of life,
> This necessary waste of flesh and blood.
> . . .
> The chyle to blood; the foaming purple tide
> To liquors, which through finer arteries
> To different parts their winding course pursue;
> . . .
> Half subtilized to chyle, the liquid food
> Readiest obeys the assimilating powers;

A splendid narrative on how and why the body needs food. The next few sections move on to the food itself and the problems of over, and under, nutrition and notes that 'Not all the culinary arts can tame, to wholesome food, the abominable growth of rest and gluttony.' So choose your diet correctly and lead an active life. He decides not to set out the various powers of individual foods as that would take too long. He does however discuss the 'fiery foods of Ind' as well as the moist melon and the pale cucumber, and the herbs and flowers which can be eaten. In addition there is the grape, the orange, the coco and ananas (pineapples) to be had. But there is a down side to all this food:

> Voluptuous Man
> Is by superior faculties misled:
> Misled from pleasure even in the quest for joy.
> Sated with nature's boons, what thousands seek,
> With dishes tortured from their native taste,
> And add variety to spurn beyond
> Its wiser will the jaded appetite!

And then a key verse:

> Is this for pleasure? Learn a juster taste
> and know, that temperance is true luxury
> Or is it pride? Pursue some nobler aim.

This sentiment is then expanded. Get rid of those parasites on your staff who 'praise for hire' and look after those who really need help from the money you would save by eating without excess: the sick, the famished, the cold, young people ('a youth of genius, whose neglected bloom unfostered sickens in barren shade'). And finally the task ahead about which we are now told:

> There are, while human miseries abound,
> A thousand ways to waste superfluous wealth,
> Without one fool or flatterer at your board,
> Without one hour of sickness or disgust.

This is a clear plea to help others if you are wealthy, and have plenty to eat. The morality of overeating is challenged.

At the opposite end a hermit's diet is needlessly severe in contrast to the 'Gross riot which treasures up a wealthy fund of plagues.' So is there a middle way?

> Learn temperance, friends; and hear without disdain
> The choice of water. Thus the Coan sage
> Opin'd and thus the learned of every school.

This is a reference to Hippocrates (the Coan sage) and to the importance of choosing water over alcohol.

Conclusion

Current interest in diet and obesity is reflected in this 18th-century poem. The problems are all well explored, and the solutions, eating wisely and taking exercise are clearly identified. Not much is new as we shall see in the next section!

Book III: Exercise

The book begins with a case study of the gardener:

> Behold the labourer of the glebe, who toils
> In dust, in rain, in cold and sultry skies:
> Save but the grain from mildews and the flood
> Nought anxious he what sickly stars ascend.
> He knows no laws by Esculapius given;
> He studies none. Yet him nor midnight fogs
> Infest, nor those envenom'd shafts that fly
> When rabid Sirius fires the autumnal noon.
> His habit pure with plain and temperate meals,
> Robust with labour, and by custom steel'd
> To every casualty of varied life.
> Serene he bears the peevish eastern blast,
> And uninfected breathes the mortal south.

The moral of this scenario is clear.

> Such the reward of rude and sober life;
> Of labour such. By health the peasant's toil
> Is well repaid.

It is this combination which has been responsible for Rome's unconquered legions and left them 'Unhurt on every soil.' So the rallying cry is 'Toil and be strong. By toil the flaccid nerves grow firm and gain more compacted tone.' So take vigorous walks, climb mountains, or chase deer. But if you get breathless and exceed your strength, choose something less tiring, but not less pleasant. Fishing, for example: choose a good river, the Stafford, the Eden, the Esk or the Liddel, this latter being the Border's river Armstrong knew best. Here the narrator identifies a number of ways in which in which physical exercise can help improve health:

> Whatever you study, in whatever you sweat,
> indulge your taste.

Some love the manly foils
The tennis some; and some the graceful dance.
Others more hardy, range the purple heath
Or naked stubble; where from field to field
The sounding coveys urge their labouring flight;
Eager amidst the rising cloud to pour
The guns unerring thunder: and there are
Whom still the meed (prize) of the green archer charms.
He chuses best, whose labour entertains
His vacant fancy most: the toil you hate
Fatigues you soon, and scarce improves your limbs.

He describes the range of sports on offer, with the clear injunction at the end that you must enjoy what you do, or you will soon tire and get little gain from the exercise. So how should we begin, assuming we need some help to get fit?

Begin with gentle toils; and, as your nerves
Grow firm, to hardier by just steps aspire.
The prudent, even in every modest walk
At first but saunter; and by slow degrees
Increase their pace.

Take it gently at first, because you might regret it.

When all at once from indolence to toil
You spring, the fibres by the hasty shock
Are tir'd and cracked, before their unctuous coats
Can pour the lubricating balm.
Besides, collected in the passive veins
The purple mass a sudden torrent rolls,
O'erpowers the heart, and deluges the lungs
With dangerous inundation: oft the source
Of fatal woes; a cough that foams with blood
Asthma, and seller Peripneumony, (inflammation of the lungs)
Or the slow minings of the hectic fire.

This is a clear description of what might happen including heart failure with coughing up blood and the circulation overpowered. There follows other bits of advice on how to avoid injury. There is much we still do not know, and must learn:

> But there are secrets which who knows not now
> Must, ere he reach them, climb the heapy Alps
> Of Science; and devote seven years of toil.

In common with other medical literature in the 18th century, baths, both hot and cold, are recommended. Here is one such recommendation:

> Plunge thrice a day, and in the tepid wave
> Untwist their stubborn pores: that full and free
> Th' evaporation thro' the softened skin
> May bear proportion to the swelling blood.
> So shall they 'scape the fevers rapid flames;
> So fell untainted the hot breath of hell.

The plunge proposed as a method of managing fevers and if pain is an issue, there is a warning about its treatment and the dangers of its treatment:

> Besides, the powerful remedies of pain
> (Since pain in spite of all our care will come)
> Should never with your prosperous days of health
> Grow too familiar: for by frequent use
> The strongest medicines lose their healing power,
> And even the surest poisons theirs to kill.

This is a clear statement of the dangers of taking pain killing drugs and their long-term consequences.

The poem then takes a different tone and covers the problems of insomnia. This includes a discussion on the hard mattress used. The weather and the seasons then feature with a statement on the diseases which occur at different times of the year:

> I in prophetic numbers could unfold
> The omens of the year: what seasons teem
> With what disease; what the humid South
> Prepares, and what the daemon of the East:

There is a salutary reminder that 'For want of timely care, millions have died of medicable wounds.'

This section of the poem ends with a description of the plague which came to England as the Plantagenets fell at Bosworth's fields and:

> Another plague or more gigantic arm
> Arose, a monster never known before
> Reared from Cocytus its portentous head
> This rapid fury not, like other pests
> Pursued a gradual course, but in a day
> Rushed as a storm o'er half the astonished isle
> And strewed with sudden carcases the land.

Death was everywhere (hence the reference to Cocytus the River of Wailing in Greek Mythology), and the symptoms vividly described. It finishes with despair,

> 'Twas all the business then
> To tend the sick, and in their turn to die
> In heaps they fell: and oft one bed, they say,
> The sickening, dying and the dead contained.

There is a plea that nothing worse will happen. 'Enough abroad, enough at home / has Albion bled.' is the cry. 'Her bravest sons, keen for the fight, have died / the death of cowards and of common men: / sunk void of wounds, and fallen without renown'. The poem then moves on, 'But from these views the weeping muses turn, and other themes invite my wandering song.'

Book IV: The Passions

Having covered air, diet, exercise (and much else) Armstrong considers the passions. He makes the important point:

> What good, what evil from ourselves proceeds
> And how the subtle Principle within
> Inspires our health, or mines with strange decay
> The passive body.

How we feel, and how our emotions rule our lives and can affect our health, is also relevant:

> By its own toil the gross corporeal frame
> Fatigues, extenuates, or destroys itself
> Nor less the labours of the mind corrode
> The solid fabric:

The influence of the mind on health is emphasised. In Armstrong's view this includes study, discontent, care, love without hope, hate without revenge, fear, jealousy, and fatigue of the soul. Such emotions can lead to depression:

> Hence the lean gloom that Melancholy wears
> The Lover's paleness; and the sallow hue
> Of Envy, Jealousy; the meagre stare
> Of sore Revenge: the cancer'd body hence
> Betrays each fretful motion of the mind.

The pedant working night and day, eating coarse food, sinks into lethargy before his time and dies of dropsy. And there is a further warning for scholars,

> But may nor the thirst of fame
> Nor love of knowledge, urge you to fatigue
> With constant drudgery the liberal soul.

Toy with your books: and, as the various fits
Of humour seize you, from Philosophy
To Fable shift; from serious Antonine
To Rabelais' ravings, and from prose to song.

For those looking for help, it's all about balance:

'Tis the great art of life to manage well
The restless mind. For ever on pursuit
Of knowledge bent, it staves the grosser powers:
Quite unemployed, against its own repose
It turns its fatal edge, and sharper pangs
Than what the body knows embitter life.
Chiefly with solitude, sad nurse of Care,
To sickly musing gives the pensive mind.
There madness enters.

So get out and about and 'seek the cheerful haunts of men, and mingle with the bustling crowd . . . or join the caravan in quest of scenes new to your eyes.' Watch out for alcohol, port, champagne, virgin wine, burgundy or the 'fresh fragrant vintage of the Rhine: and wish that heaven from mortals had withheld the grape, and all intoxicating bowls.'

Happiness is then discussed, 'How to live happiest; how to avoid the pains, the disappointments, and the disgusts of those who would in pleasure all their hours employ.' He tells the story of a wise old man and how happiness is our common pursuit. It will not be found however in seeking pleasure, of whatever sort. The answer is virtue:

Virtue (for mere Good-nature is a fool)
Is sense and spirit with humanity
Tis sometimes angry, and its frown confounds;
Tis even vindictive, but in vengeance just

This is what makes prosperity worth while, it gives peace and shelter in adversity, and on this foundation you can build your fame defying envy and the gloss of fortune and 'the praise that's worth ambition is attained by sense alone, and dignity of mind.' This culminates in a striking section on what it's all about:

> Virtue, the strength and beauty of the soul
> Is the best gift of heaven: a happiness
> That even above the smiles and frowns of fate
> Exalts great Natures favourites: a wealth
> that ne'er encumbers, nor to baser hands
> can be transferred; it is the only good
> man justly boasts of, or can call his own.

The author must move on, 'Formed in the School of Paeon (the Physician of the Olympian Gods), I relate what passions hurt the body, what improve, avoid them, or invite them, as you may.' He makes the point that the most vital thing that mortals feel is hope 'the life blood of the soul. It pleases and it lasts . . . Our greatest good, and what we least can spare is Hope; the last of all our evils is fear.' Other things may matter, love, beauty, these may add 'bloom to health' but they can go wrong. 'Some have died for love; and some run mad; and some with desperate hand themselves have slain.'

Nor should you let luxury or a quest for renown make you do things you might regret. You will become a ghost of what you were, languid melancholy and gaunt. Disease will haunt you and age creep on. Anger, envy, grief, rage, these can cause apoplexy or a fever:

> As is the passion such is still the Pain
> The body feels; or chronic or acute
> And oft a sudden storm at once o'erpowers
> The life, or gives you reason to the winds.
> Such fates attend the rash alarm of Fear,
> And sudden Grief, and Rage and sudden Joy.

There is advice too about anger management:

> While Choler works, good friend, you may be wrong;
> Distrust yourself, and sleep before you fight.

'Tis not too late tomorrow to be brave;
If honour bids, tomorrow kill or die
But calm advice against a raging fit
Avails too little;

However there is a solution:

There is a Charm, a Power, that sways the breast;
Bids every Passion revel or be still
Inspires with Rage, or all your Cares dissolves;
Can sooth Distraction, and almost Despair.
That power is Music: far beyond the stretch
Or those unmeaning warblers on the stage;

And the climax of the poem, in the last few lines, summarises the message:

Music exalts each Joy, allays each Grief
Expels Diseases, softens every Pain,
Subdues the rage of Poison, and the Plague;
And hence the wise of ancient days ador'd
One Power of Physic, Melody, and Song.

Some reflections

This is a remarkable and very contemporary poem. It sets out some of the determinants of health and in particular emphasises the relevance of the 'passions' in influencing well-being and quality of life. The final reference to the role of music picks up a very current theme linking the arts to health.

One interesting question to ask is how would such a poem be written now? Setting aside some of the language issues, the main determinants are represented though in a modern context they would be expanded. For example the 'Book on Air' would certainly have covered a wider range of environmental issues; water quality, chemicals, radiation, and health and safety.

The 'Book on Diet' would again have been developed to include other lifestyle issues such as tobacco, drugs and alcohol, though this is covered later to some extent. It might also have been merged with the 'Book on Exercise'. The 'Book on Passions' is of particular interest. This topic, the role of the emotions in determining health is much less talked about at present and it provides a stimulus to re-think this subject.

Finally, there is no mention of the genetic basis for health and illness, and this is perhaps not surprising. Nor is there any real discussion on the role of the health service or carers in improving health, again for very obvious reasons. Perhaps the challenge is to write a 21st-century version of *The Art of Preserving Health*.

Notes

1   John Armstrong, *The Art of Preserving Health*, 4 vols (London: T Davies, 1774), I, ll. 1–5.

2   Adam Budd, *John Armstrong's The Art of Preserving Health* (Farnham: Ashgate, 2011).

3   M. J. Dobson, 'History of Malaria in England', *Journal of the Royal Society of Medicine*, 82 (1989), 3–7.

CHAPTER 11

Further writing from the 18th century

> When agues shake, or fevers raise a flame,
> Let your physician be a man of fame
> Of well-known learning, and in good respect
> For prudence, honour, and a mind erect.
>
> Allan Ramsay

This chapter brings together a number of authors from the 18th century who have written poems, novels and songs with a health and well-being theme. They range widely, but show the depth and spread of material from this time in Scottish culture and heritage.

William Hamilton of Gilbertfield (c1665–1751)

William Hamilton was a retired army lieutenant, who had strong links with Allan Ramsay with whom he corresponded in verse. It was Hamilton's edition of *Blind Harry's Wallace* which was so important to Robert Burns. Hamilton wrote a reflective poem entitled 'The last dying words of Bonny Heck, a famous grey-hound in the shire of Fife' (1706)[1]

Bonny Heck is a famous grey hound, the best around but now he must be 'hing by the neck' just for being old:

> Alas, alas, quo bonny Heck,
> On former days when I reflect!
> I was a dog in much respect
> For doughty Deed:
> But now I must hing by the neck
> Without rameed.

He's been the best, but no one will stand up for him now:

> But now, good Sirs, this day is lost
> The best dog in the East Nook Coast,
> For never ane durst Brag not Boast
> Me, for their neck
> But now I must yield up the ghost
> Quo' bonnie heck

However, this is not because 'I'm a cripple, auld and lame' but for other reasons. Even though he could beat the hare and be in the front of the race. He has done nothing wrong, he is just old and must be put down. His one joy is that he has puppies and they will keep his memory alive when he is gone.

> But if my puppies, ance were ready
> Which I got on a bonny lady
> They'l be baith Clever, Keen and Beddy
> And ne'er neglect
> To clink it like their ancient Daddy
> The famous Heck.

This poem was the inspiration for another word of advice, this time the advice of 'Lucky Spence' from Allan Ramsay. But 'Bonny Heck' also has remarkably modern connotations in the current debates and ethical issues on death and dying.

Allan Ramsay (1686–1758)

Allan Ramsay was born in Leadhills in Lanarkshire, and educated at the parish school in Crawford. He moved to Edinburgh in 1701 and apprenticed to a wig maker, eventually setting up shop himself in the High Street. He married in 1712 and had six children, his eldest being Allan Ramsay the portrait painter. He became a member of the Easy Club taking the names Isaac Bickerstaff and later Gawin Douglas. He began publishing and writing verse and moved to the Luckenbooths, opened a circulating library (the first in Scotland) and developed his business as a bookseller.

Three poems are of particular interest in relation to literature and health, the first being his own first poem, 'To the Memory of Dr Archibald Pitcairne'.[2] Pitcairne had died in October 1713 and had a reputation for patriotism which may have appealed to members of the Easy Club. He was a very distinguished Edinburgh physician, who had founded the College of Physicians in Edinburgh and maintained a strong link to Leiden in Holland, then the centre of the medical world, which Edinburgh was to overtake later in the century. The poem itself says little about medicine or health but does reflect the patriotism and the idea of Scottish independence, remembering that the Union of Parliaments in 1707 was just a few years away:

> O Gods! Is the Great Soul of SCOTLAND fled;
> Or does She Dream on some dark drowsy bed.
> Will she not rise to gain Her Old Renown,
> And show She wears an Independent Crown.

There is also an important reference to Scotland's role in learning, which was about to come to fullness in the 18th century Enlightenment.

> And those, who for their learning had their name,
> Wrote in the endless bright records of fame.

The second poem is 'Lucky Spence's Last Advice' (1718) the tale of a dying prostitute who gives her advice to her followers.[3] It has its basis in the 'Dying words of Bonny Heck.' She knows she is dying and after asking for a gill dispenses her thoughts, much of which is directed to getting as much money from her patrons, as well as giving to them, the 'pox'. Her advice is clear to her acolytes about their clients:

> When he's asleep then dive and catch
> His ready cash, his rings and watch;
> And gin he takes to light his match
> At your spunk-box.

Ne'er stand to let the fumbling wretch
E'en take the pox

She then has words for the men who are good to her and her girls, and those
who are bad, don't pay and drink too much. It ends with a forecast on their
health.

My benison come on good doers
Who spend their cash on bawds and whores
May they never want the wale of cures
For a sair snout
Foul fa' the quacks wha that fire smoors
And puts nae out.

My malison light ilka day
On them that drink and dinna pay
But tak a snack and rin way
May 't be their hap
Never to want a gonorrhoea
Or rotten clap.

The poem shows significant understanding of venereal disease with a reference to 'sair snout' a sign of syphilis, and that the many treatments available
are not effective. In a subsequent poem (Health) Ramsay refers to the use of
mercury in treatment, the only remedy available until the advent of antibiotics in the mid-20th century.

The final poem of Ramsay's is one on 'Health' inscribed to the Earl of
Stair and written in 1724.[4] It presents, in a series of vignettes, the determinants of good health and bad health, contrasts them, and gives suggestions
for the way forward.

The first vignette considers a man with fine clothes, carried in his chair
to dine and who eats and drinks well. His liver is inflamed, and he coughs
and wheezes but he cannot smile. His riches and his wealth can do nothing
to help. Even his cook cannot tempt him to eat. It is the same with the rake,
all his pleasures have gone while he sweats and turns, and starts and raves:

> How mad's that man, pushed by his passions wild
> Who's of his greatest happiness beguiled
> Who seems, whate'er he says, by actions low
> To court disease, our pleasure's greatest foe.

Seeking pleasure is not the way to health, and indeed can bring ill health.

Food is the next subject to be tackled and there follows a list of exotic foodstuffs, and then the consequences of overindulgence:

> Of them who eat the dangerous repast
> Until the feeble stomach's over crammed
> The fibre weakened and the blood enflam'd
> What aching heads, what spleen and drowsy eyes
> From undigested crudities arise!

And then the conclusion to this part of the poem, 'Luxurious man! Altho' thou art blest with wealth / Why should thou use it to destroy thy health?' The dangers of a luxurious life, of overeating and of lack of exercise are clearly illustrated.

To improve your health you should copy Mellantius. Don't eat or drink too much, and only when you are hungry or thirsty.

It also does not help to have the wrong attitude to life. Take Grumaldo. He works too hard, toils all day, is exhausted and full of envy. His life is joyless and:

> Meagre disease and easy passage finds
> Where joy's debarred, in such corroded minds
> Such take no care the springs of life to save
> Neglect their health, and quickly fill the grave.

Myrtil is quite different:

> Unlike gay Myrtil, who, with cheerful air
> Less envious, tho' less rich, no slave to care
> Thinks what he has enough, and scorns to fret
>
> . . .

155

Thus envy finds no access to his breast
To sour his gen'rous joy, or break his rest
He studies to do actions just and kind
Which with the best reflections cheer the mind;

And then the message:

Which is the first preservative of health,
To be preferred to grandeur, pride and wealth
Let all who would pretend to common sense
'Gainst pride and envy still be on defence
Who love their health, nor would their joys control
Let them ne'er nurse such furies in their soul

Phimos shows another side of illness, a man laden with vile diseases purchased from women who look unwell; the consequence, venereal disease, and especially syphilis. We are told of Phimos:

He grasps the blasted shadows of the fair
Whose sickly look, vile breath and falling hair
The flagged embrace and mercenary squeeze
The tangs of guilt, and terrors of disease
Might warn him to beware, if wild desire
Had not set all his thoughtless soul on fire
O poor mistaken youth! To drain thy purse
To gain the most malignant human curse!
Think in thy flannel, and mercurial dose
And future pains to save thy nerve and nose.

This is a wonderful description of syphilis and the consequences, together with the reference to treatment with mercury:

How frightful is the loss, and the disgrace
When it destroys the beauties of the face!
When the arch nose in rotten ruin lies
And all the venom flames around the eyes;

When the uvula has got its mortal wound
And tongue and lips form words without a sound
When hair drops off, and bones corrupt and bare
Through ulcerated tags of muscles stare.

This is a real description of the disease, not from the textbooks but from regularly seeing people who have been infected. It suggests that the disease is common and readily recognised.

Good marriage and bad marriage are then described, and the value of a happy marriage clearly set out:

To him has many a winter wedded wife
Appears the greatest solace of his life
He views his offspring with indulgent love
Who his superior conduct all approve.
Smooth glide his hours; at fifty he's less old
Than some who have not half the numbers told
The cheering glass he with right friends can share
But shuns the deep debauch with care
His sleeps are sound, he sees the morning rise
And lifts his face with pleasure to the skies.

The problems with over indulging in wine are then described. If only they could stop. 'Fools should not drink, I own, who still wish more / And know not when 'tis proper to give o'er.' The sloth 'too oft the child of wealth' then comes under examination. Ramsay gives splendid description of the weak and feeble person who sits all day by the fire in his easy chair, and even when he plays cards, you must deal, because it causes too much pain to deal the cards himself. And at the end,

Thus does the sluggard health and vigour waste
With heavy indolence, till, at the last
Sciatica, jaundice, dropsy or the stone
Alternate makes the lazy lubbard groan.

This explicit description of the inactive life is then compared to that of the active Hilaris, who likes to take exercise and walk and bound through the countryside. The poem gives a vivid description of the exercise available at the time. Here Ramsay sets out what the athlete enjoys:

> The race delights him, horses are his care,
> And a stout ambling pad his easiest chair
> Sometimes, to firm his nerves, he'll plunge the deep
> And with expanded arms the billows sweep:
> Then on the links, or on the estler walls
> He drives the gowff, or strikes the tennis-balls.
> From ice with pleasure he can brush the snow
> And run rejoicing with his curling throw;
> Or send the whizzing arrow from the string
> A manly game, which by itself I sing.

But things can go too far and taken to excess. That can be just as bad:

> Here let no youth, extravagantly given
> Who values neither gold, nor health, nor Heaven
> Think that our song encourages the crime
> Of setting deep, or wasting too much time
> On furious game, which makes the passions boil,
> And the fair mean of health a weak'ning toil,
> By violence excessive, or the pain
> Which ruined losers ever must sustain.

And when illness strikes, what then?

> But when these ills intrude, do what we will
> Then hope for health from Clerk's approved skill
> To such, well seen in natures darker laws,
> That for disorders can assign a cause;
> Who knows the virtues of salubrious plants,
> And what each different constitution wants,

Apply for health—But shun the vagrant quack
Who gulls the crowd with Andrew's comic clack;
Or him that charges gazettes with his bills,
His anodynes, elixirs, tinctures, pills,
Who rarely ever cures, but often kills.
Nor trust thy life to the old woman's charms,
Who binds with knotted tape thy legs or arms
Which they pretend will purple fevers cool,
And thus impose on some believing fool.

An interesting comment here on the need to identify the cause of illness and to know the various plants which might help to heal. So which kind of person do you need to help the healing process?

When agues shake, or fevers raise a flame,
Let your physician be a man of fame
Of well-known learning, and in good respect
For prudence, honour, and a mind erect.
Not scrimply save from what's to merit due;
He saves your whole estate who succours you.

You need someone who has the learning, but who also has values and who is well respected. Finally, Ramsay notes the importance of climate on health. He contrasts Lapland with the heat of Africa and the fevers which occur, and the ravenous beasts and serpents. The comment on ague-malaria has already been discussed. In Africa 'Health must be here a stranger, where the rage / Of fev'rish beams forbids a lengthen'd age.'

He discusses the Dutch and the Spanish climates but blesses 'the Queen of Isles' which is a healthful place, which is where he wants to stay. This is a remarkable poem, very forward thinking and modern, identifying the key determinants of health. These, as will be seen recur again and again, they have not just been discovered but have been recognised for centuries.

- Plenty of exercise, but not too much
- Adequate food, but not too much

- No drinking to excess
- Avoidance of venereal disease
- No bad feelings of envy or pride, but joy in the little things
- A pleasant environment
- A happy marriage
- And a good doctor to help

Each of these a clear link to the determinants of health set out at the introduction of this book; social and economic factors, lifestyle, environment,
and medical care. There is little on the other hand about the causes of
disease, or genetic issues, these would need to wait another two centuries
to be considered.

Finally from Ramsay a few lines from 'The Gentle Shepherd'[5] a pastoral
poem about love, realtionships and work. In this single line he summarises
his thoughts on quality of life:

> He that has just enough can soundly sleep.

This is a very succint way of encapsulating how to sleep well and have a good
quality of life.

His thoughts on education in 'The Gentle Shepherd' are also worth
noting. Peggy notes about her shepherd lover:

> Ilk day that he's alane upon the hill,
> He reads fell books that teach him meikle skill

And in the words of Sir William, his master, about the shepherd:

> He answered well; and much ye glad my ear
> When such accounts I of my shepherd hear.
> Reading such books can raise a peasant's mind
> Above a lord's that is not thus inclin'd.

This emphasises the importance the ability of even the most lowly to benefit from and to love reading and learning.

Robert Blair (1699–1746)

Robert Blair was born in Edinburgh and educated at the university there, and in Holland. Blair published only three poems and his most famous is 'The Grave' (1743), and is particularly noted for the engravings by William Blake in 1808.[6] It is a genre of poem which reflects the interest in death and the graveyard. He describes the school boy and new-made widow in the dark space between the tombs. Anticipating Tam o' Shanter, the schoolboy as he moves through the graveyard:

> Full fast he flies, and dare not look behind him
> Till, out of breath, he overtakes his fellows
> Who gather round and wonder at the tale
> Of horrid apparition tall and ghastly
> That walks at dead of night, or takes his stand
> O'er some new-opened grave; and (strange to tell!)
> Evanishes at crowing of the cock.

There is a fascination with death and the pain of leaving and loss. Of happiness, of things not said and joys departed.

> . . . Oh! Then the longest summer's day
> Seem'd too, too much in haste; still the full heart
> Had not imparted half; t'was happiness
> Too exquisite to last. Of joys departed,
> Not to return, how painful the remembrance!

Those bereaved can understand such sentiments, and for those caring for them, remembrance, and the joys which have been, can be comforting.

The Reverend John Skinner (1721–1807)

John Skinner was born in Aberdeenshire and educated at Marischal College in Aberdeen. He joined the Scottish Episcopal Church and became minister of Longside, near Linshart. He wrote an *Ecclesiastical History of Scotland* (1788), but is most famous for 'Tullochgorum' (1769) a song which Burns described as the 'best Scotch Song ever Scotland saw.'[7] They had a fascinating correspondence. It was suggested that Skinner might write the words to go with the air 'The Reel o' Tullochgorum' by Mrs Montgomery from Ellon. It covers the good things in life, and the bad things, all in praise of the 'Reel o' Tullochgorum'. This verse sets out the good life in a benefaction:

> May choicest blessings aye attend
> Each honest, open-hearted friend
> And calm and quiet be his end
>   And a' that's good watch o'er him
> May peace and plenty be his lot,
>   Peace and plenty, peace and plenty,
>   Peace and plenty be his lot
>   And dainties a great store o' them
> May peace and plenty be his lot,
> Unstain'd by any vicious spot
> And may he never wish a groat,
>   That's fond of Tullochgorum.

However, if you are sullen and discontented:

> But for the sullen frumpish fool,
> That loves to be oppression's tool
> May envy gnaw his rotten soul,
>   And discontent devour him
> May dool and sorrow be his chance, (woe)
>   Dool and sorrow, dool and sorrow
>   Dool and sorrow be his chance
>   And nane say, "wae's me" for him!

May dool and sorrow be his chance
Wi' a' the ills that come frae France
Wha e'er he be that winna dance,
    The Reel of Tullochgorum.

Much in the style of other writers it praises those who are honest, open-hearted and who have a good word for everyone.

Henry Mackenzie (1745–1835)

Mackenzie was born in Edinburgh and educated there at the high school and university. While based in that city he was admitted as an Attorney in the Court of Exchequer and made frequent visits to London. He wrote many works, but the novel which is best remembered is *The Man of Feeling* written in 1771, and it was an immediate success.[8] He was politically active and wrote extensively. His review of Burns' poems was where Burns was first called 'this heaven-taught ploughman'. *The Man of Feeling* is a fascinating read, even today, particularly as the 'Index of Tears' (which first appeared in 1886) sets out how often tears were used in the text. Of interest to the medical context was a visit made to Bedlam in Moorfields in London:

Of those things called sights in London, which every stranger is supposed desirous to see, Bedlam is one. To that place therefore, an acquaintance of Harley's, after having accompanied him to several other shows, proposed a visit. Harley objected to it, 'because,' he said, 'I think it an inhuman practice to expose the greatest misery with which our nature is afflicted, to every idle visitant who can afford a trifling perquisite to the keeper; especially as it is a distress which the humane must see with the painful reflection, that it is not in their power to alleviate it.' He was overpowered however by the solicitations of his friend, and other persons of the party (amongst whom were several ladies); and they went in a body to Moorfields.

Their conductor led them first to the dismal mansions of those who are in the most horrid state of incurable madness. The clanking of chains, the wildness of their cries, and the imprecations which some of them uttered, formed a scene so inexpressible shocking, Harley and his companions, especially the female part of them, begged their guide to return

It would be impossible today to have such a visiting party to a hospital, never mind an asylum, just to give them something to do on a dull afternoon. The description, limited as it is, is distressing and it is no wonder that the party wanted to move on. Such a visit, and the ethical implications of it, would surely not be possible in the 21st century.

Mac Mhaighstir Alasdair

Mac Mhaighstir Alasdair was a Baillie on Canna and in 1751 he published a small book of Gaelic verse.[9] The poems have been commented on by John Lorne Campbell.[10] It contains a particularly interesting poem on venereal disease in Ardnamurchan, perhaps brought to Strontian by English workers in the York Company's lead mines. The language, in Campbell's words is obscene but it is an important contribution and requires further study and analysis.[11]

Postscript

JAMES BEATTIE (1735–1803) was a distinguished Professor of Moral Philosophy in Aberdeen, and referred to in Burns' poems. He had a particular interest in commonsense philosophy, and he published widely on that subject. Like many others he saw a conflict in the use of Scots for writing, as opposed to 'English'. As a result he wrote a Treatise on *Scoticisms, arranged in alphabetical order designed to correct improprieties of speech and writing.*[12] (1797) It is a collection of Scots words and sayings and how to correct them and make them understandable to those South of the border. For example, from a very long list:

> Anent: with regard to or concerning.
> Amissing: missing
> I asked at him: I asked him[13]

This tension is reflected in the varying language used by writers such as Ramsay and Burns and has been the subject of much discussion and debate. The topic is of particular relevance to this book as much of the content relates to the language used and the meaning of the terms employed by the writers which gives a particularly Scottish focus to their works.

Notes

1 William Hamilton of Gilbertfield, 'The Last Dying Words of Bonny Heck, a Famous Grey-hound in the Shire of Fife', in Christopher MacLachlan, ed., *Before Burns: Eighteenth-Century Scottish Poetry* (Edinburgh: Canongate Classics, 2002), pp. 15–17.

2 Allan Ramsay, 'A Poem to the Memory of Alexander Pitcairne' (1713), in *The Bibliotheck*, 7 (1979), 153–160.

3 'Lucky Spence's Last Advice', in MacLachlan, *Before Burns*, pp. 25–9.

4 'Health', in *The Poems of Allan Ramsay*, 2 vols (Paisley: Alex Gardner, 1877), I, pp. 69–81.

5 Ramsay, *Gentle Shepherd,* p. 17 line 1.

6 Robert Blair, *The Grave* (London: Scatcherd and Whitaker, 1747).

7 *Lindsay, The Burns Encyclopedia*, p. 334. and John Skinner, 'Tullochgorum', in MacLachlan, *Before Burns*, pp. 185–7.

8 Henry Mackenzie, *The Man of Feeling*, ed. Brian Vickers (Oxford: Oxford University Press, 1987).

9 Alexander MacDonald, Baillie of Canna, *The Resurrection of the Ancient Scottish Language, or the New Highland Songster* (Edinburgh: [n.pub], 1751).

10 J.L. Campbell, *Canna: The Story of a Hebridean Island*, 3rd ed. (Oxford: Oxford University Press, 1994).

11 I am grateful to the preliminary work of Dr Sheila Kidd on this poem and the encouragement of Dr Hugh Cheape.

12 James Beattie, *Scoticisms, arranged in alphabetical order designed to correct improprieties of speech and writing* (Edinburgh: William Creech, 1797).

13 Ibid, p. 1.

CHAPTER 12

The Industrial Revolution and the first real steps for change.

The nineteenth century in Scotland

Heave awa lads I'm no deid yet!

The 19th century was a period of significant change in medicine, science and in society. Scotland was part of major international events such as the Napoleonic wars, and the Crimean war, together with the movement of large numbers of Scots across the world.

In terms of medicine there were several major advances that changed the way in which patients were treated and gave new hope for the future. Two of these were initiated in Scotland. The first was anaesthesia, where in Edinburgh James Young Simpson was the first to use the gas chloroform in childbirth. In addition this allowed major surgical procedures to be carried out under optimal conditions. The conditions before the introduction of anaesthesia are well described in a short story by Dr John Brown, *Rab and his Friends* (1859) which will be discussed later. The second major advance was in antiseptic surgery, this time in Glasgow by Joseph Lister. Again this allowed further surgical developments and new procedures.

At the same time medicine was advancing on other fronts. The knowledge of the body grew through developments in anatomy and physiology, though sometimes the methods used were less than appropriate. It was the era of the resurrectionists and the body snatchers, and the infamous Robert Knox. A key part of the progress was in pathology and bacteriology, using microscopy for example, and this led to the identification of what caused disease and how it could be reversed. Much of this was done in Germany, and Rudolf Virchow and Robert Koch (who identified the bacterium which

166

caused tuberculosis) pioneered this work closely involved with scientists in Scotland. Pasteur in Paris also continued the identification of the organisms which caused the disease and opened the way for new methods of treatment, though it would be the 20th century before antibiotics were discovered. Claude Bernard in France began the process of greater understanding of the physiology of the chemistry of the body. Darwin's *The Origin of the Species* (1859) provided a new way of thinking about man and his place in nature.

In surgery new methods began to be developed including the treatment of breast cancer by removing the ovaries, pioneered by Sir George Beatson in 1896 in Glasgow and in new methods of operating on the stomach and bowel by Theodore Billroth in Germany. Again in Glasgow there were pioneering operations on the brain and chest by Sir William Macewen. By the turn of the century Marie Curie had discovered radium and a new treatment for cancer, and William Conrad Rontgen had shown the first X-ray, first used in Scotland by Dr MacIntyre at the Royal Infirmary in Glasgow. All of these were developed further in the 20th century

Hospitals and the provision of health care changed considerably and in many of the narratives, to be described, the facilities were primitive. It was difficult to find a doctor, to pay for one and to know whether or not the individual was qualified. All of this began to change with the advent of Voluntary Hospitals, medical missions, and the beginnings of a public health service.

The Medical Act of 1858 was a significant development with the introduction of a register of all qualified doctors, following on from the Apothecaries Act of 1815. The General Medical Council (GMC) was set up, which maintained this register and established criteria for quality in medical practice. Medical education began to change and in both Edinburgh and Glasgow there were a number of extra-mural schools. The curriculum expanded, subject to approval by the GMC. The clinical method and the stethoscope were introduced from France, and the now standard methods of history taking, inspection, palpation, percussion and auscultation became routine. By the end of the century women were being admitted to medical school. There was a new interest in medical societies, many of which were set up in the 19th century, and the *British Medical Journal* and the *Lancet* began publishing.

Public health measures were gradually introduced, and the first Medical Officer of Health in Scotland was appointed in Edinburgh in 1862 following the collapse of a tenement in the High Street. The quotation at the head of this chapter is engraved above a close in the High Street in Edinburgh where a young boy survived and was pulled out. Legislation, including the Poor Law Amendment Act of 1845, became an important way of dealing with social issues and a wide range of charities were set up to deal with the homeless and the orphaned. There were also significant public movements, generally driven by religious groups, who aimed to deal with the social problems of the times, such as prostitution, crime and alcohol abuse. Several of the matters raised later, deal with such issues. The Temperance Movement was especially strong, with organisations such as the Band of Hope actively promoting abstinence in schools and at public events. Mental health hospitals were established, often to deal with the relatives of those who could afford it, and were large dark places with extensive grounds, some of which are still in use. It was also an era of great medical missionaries such as David Livingstone (1813–1873), with his work in Africa.

There were some remarkable ventures such as the development at New Lanark, mentioned earlier, begun in 1785 by Robert Owen, a place where work, education and religion would produce a new type of community. Thomas Chalmers (1780–1847), a Church of Scotland minister, attacked the problem of poverty in his writings and actions and these were replicated in mission and voluntary groups across the country. He had moved to Glasgow, to the Tron Church in the centre of town, but in 1819 moved to St John's in the Carlton, a particularly poor place, where he carried out innovative work to alleviate the squalor and poverty around him. The disruption of the Church of Scotland in 1843 added another dimension to this. The role of the working classes in this period is well set out in Thomas Johnston's book, *The History of the Working Classes in Scotland* (1920).[1]

It was also a time of significant constitutional change with the Reform Act 1884, the Crofters Commission of 1886 and the Chartism Movement seeking male suffrage, secret ballots, equal electoral districts, paid MPs and abolition of property qualifications. The Education Act of 1867 provided another important way forward. There was the birth of socialism in Scotland. There was also a rise in the middle classes, people who had made substantial fortunes, much of which came back to the community in philanthropic giving.

All of this was occurring at a time of considerable social change. Its centre-piece was the Industrial Revolution which provided a huge opportunity for employment and increased wages in Scotland. The population moved from the countryside to the cities and there was a need for rapid house building and social provision. Here in the tenements were the slums, poverty and disease. Some of this was driven by changes in the land, with the clearances in the Highlands and the mass emigration to Canada, America, Australia and New Zealand, some of it forced. There was also major immigration, especially from Ireland, to swell the housing requirements of the west of Scotland. Glasgow, Greenock and Paisley all grew hugely, initially due to the cotton industry, then coal, steel and heavy engineering and shipbuilding, leaving a lasting legacy into the 20th century.

The remote areas of Scotland had different problems. For example St Kilda, a group of islands in the far north west, had very high infant mortality rates due to neonatal tetanus, and the population was subject to major infections when a boat from one of the other islands or the mainland arrived.[2]

Railways significantly changed the movement of the population, as did the impact of newspapers on local communities. Some communities sprung up around the rail network and new towns developed. In Glasgow in 1859 Queen Victoria opened the Loch Katrine Water Works and they began operation the following year. This was a very significant public health measure.

Scotland changed in other ways. Following the visit to Scotland in 1822 by King George IV and the interest of Queen Victoria in Scotland, tartan and tourism became important and the Home Rule movement began, first as the National Association for the Vindication of Scottish Rights in 1853, and then the Scottish Home Rule Association in 1886.

In the small towns and villages of Scotland during the century, and especially in the first half, there was a social structure which worked to help the community. There was the minister, the school teacher (the dominie) and the doctor, generally supported by the local landowner. They were able to identify the gifted child, generally a boy (the lad o' pairts), and ensure that they had sufficient education to get them to university. The community often clubbed together to pay fees and in most Scottish Universities there are bursaries for students from such small places. The local laird was also often very helpful in this regard.

The literature of Scotland over this period was considererable, and only a relatively small part will be covered in this section of the book. In addition to books, there was a healthy trade in magazines such as the *Edinburgh Review*, and *Blackwood's Magazine* (edited by John Wilson under the pseudonym Christopher North). These provided space for stories and poems. At this period in 1825 the world's first comic book was published as the *Glasgow Looking Glass* with illustrations of current political issues of a satirical nature.

In considering the literature of Scotland in the 19th century related to health, the discussion is set out by theme, rather than by individual authors. These themes are 'Doctors and Medical Students', 'Health, Illness and Remedies', and 'Social Conditions and Lifestyle' and they are covered in the next three chapters. In most instances the authors will be described as they appear, but some authors are covered in more than one chapter, and are thus noted at this stage.

Sir Walter Scott (1771–1832)

Only six of Scott's parents' twelve children survived infancy. Walter was born in College Wynd in Edinburgh and as a child developed poliomyelitis at eighteen months, retaining a limp all his life. He was sent to his grandfather's farm in the Borders, where he developed a taste for tales. He entered the High School in Edinburgh and then appreticed as a copy clerk in his father's practice. He met Burns as a young man of fifteen years old and subsequently qualified as an advocate. On a trip to the Lake District he met Charlotte Margaret Charpentier, proposed to her three weeks later and they were married on Christmas Eve 1797. He began to write at the age of twenty-five and his first book was linked to his love of the Scottish Borders, *The Minstrelsy of the Scottish Borders* (1802–1803). He was appointed Deputy Sherriff of the County of Selkirk. His first literary success was in poetry (*Marmion* 1808, *Lady of the Lake* 1810) and his first novel, published anonymously, was *Waverley* (1814). There then followed a whole series of romantic, historical novels which were widely read. He was always in financial difficulty and much of his writing was done to pay the bills. He bought land near Melrose and built his home, Abbotsford, there, where he died in 1832, and was buried in Dryburgh Abbey. His legacy to literature and to Scotland is enormous. In 1822 he stage-managed the visit of George IV to Edinburgh, which was a major event in which tartan and cultural history played a significant role. *The Letters of Malachi Malagrowther* (1826) published in the *Edinburgh Weekly* caused a change in Government policy and related to the ability of Scottish Banks to produce their own bank notes. This is a topic which remains of some interest.

James Hogg (1770–1835)

Hogg, sometimes known as the Ettrick Shepherd, was determined to become a poet after reading 'Tam o' Shanter' by Robert Burns. He taught himself to read and write, helped by his employer giving him access to a library. He was introduced to Sir Walter Scott who asked him to help with the publication of *The minstrelsy of the Scottish Border* (1802–1803). He had numerous poems published and several novels, the most famous of which was *The Private Memoirs and Confessions of a Justified Sinner* (1824) published anonymously. It made little critical impact at the time but has since, mainly in the 20th century, received much aclaim. Much of his work was published in magazines, such as *Blackwood's*.

John Galt (1779–1839)

Born in Irvine and brought up in Greenock, Galt left for London but his business failed so he toured the Mediterranean and Near East for two years, and met the young Byron. He moved to Canada where he founded the City of Guelph in 1827, but as a businessman was never successful. He retired to Greenock in Scotland and died in 1839. He wrote *Annals of the Parish*, but the publisher turned it down as being too local and too Scottish: it eventually appeared in print in 1821. Other books he wrote included *The Ayrshire Legatees* (1821), which proved popular. The *Provost* and the *Entail* were published in 1822 and 1823 respectively.

Robert Louis Stevenson (1850–1894)

Robert was born in Edinburgh and lived in the New Town, and died in Samoa aged 44. He suffered from ill health (a weak chest) for many years and required considerable medical treatment. Indeed the reason for his going to Samoa was because of his health. His father was a leading lighthouse engineer and this connection will be referred to later. Stevenson was educated in Edinburgh, often with private tutors and when he entered the University of Edinburgh he did his best to avoid lectures. He travelled in his early years, but his health was poor and he went to the South of France to recuperate, returning to Scotland in 1874 and to his studies, qualifying for the Scottish Bar in 1875. He never practised law. Robert met the American, Fanny Vandegrift Osbourne, who had been previously married and had three children, and they became lovers and married in 1880. He moved to San Francisco and lived in various places in Europe and in each of these required medical help. These encounters are noted in his poem 'Underwoods' which will be discussed later. Stevenson then moved to the Pacific Islands and his writing there included the *Master of Ballantrae* (1889). He purchased land in Samoa, built a house and died there in 1894. His literary output was significant and in addition to the adventure stories such as *Treasure Island* (1883), and *Kidnapped* (1886) he also wrote the mystery story *The Strange Case of Dr Jekyll and Mr Hyde* (1886). He wrote numerous poems and one of this most noted collections was *A Child's Garden of Verse* (1885) His last, unfinished, novel was *Weir of Hermiston* (1896) published after his death.

The Kailyard

The Kailyard is the name given to a group of Scottish authors, which covered the period 1888 until around 1900. The origin of the name, kail-yard or cabbage patch, is disputed and it may be related to MacLaren's use of the phrase in *Beside the Bonnie Brier Bush* (1894). 'There grows a bonnie brier bush in our kail-yard / And white are the blossoms on't in our kail-yard'.[3]Burns wrote a similar poem 'There grows a bonie brier-bush', which uses *in our kail-yard* in its first line.[4]It was a very popular genre and the main authors associated with it were J.M. Barrie, Ian MacLaren and Samuel Rutherford

Crockett. The person who did most to promote the Kailyard was William Robertson Nicoll, editor of the *BritishWeekly*, a non-conformist paper which published many of the authors' poems and stories. The poetry and stories are sentimental and while enormously popular at the time they have not had a very favourable criticism. The authors J.M. Barrie, Ian MacLaren, and George Douglas Brown have extracts from their works used in the chapters which follow.

James Matthew Barrie (1860–1937)

J.M. Barrie was born in Kirriemuir in Angus and educated in Glasgow, Forfar, Dumfries and Edinburgh University. Following his education he moved to London where he worked for a time as a journalist and met the Llewelyn Davies boys who inspired the writing of *Peter Pan*. He wrote widely and when he died he left the publishing rights of *Peter Pan* to Great Ormond Street Children's Hospital in London. He was a shy and introverted person. His first novels, *Auld Licht Idylls* (1888), *A Window in Thrums* and *The Little Minister* all reflect his background in Kirriemuir. He had significant social connections and marred Mary Ansell in 1891. He died of pneumonia, in 1937 and is buried in Kirriemuir.

Ian Maclaren (1850–1907)

Ian Maclaren was the pseudonym of the Reverend John Watson. He was born in Essex and educated in Stirling and Edinburgh University. He studied theology at New College Edinburgh and Tubingen. Watson was minister in Edinburgh, Logiealmond and Glasgow before moving to Sefton Park in Liverpool. His first stories of Scottish Rural Life were *Beside the Bonnie Briar Bush* (1894) and they were extremely popular as were his subsequent books.

William Topas McGonagall (1825–1902)

William McGonagall was born in Edinburgh of Irish parents. He moved to Dundee where he spent most of his life, where he was a weaver. He was inspired to become a poet and wrote 'The most startling incident in my life was the time I discovered myself to be a poet.'[5] McGonagall described himself as a poet and tragedian and is considered by some to be the worst poet in British history, writing over 200 poems published as a series of *Poetic Gems,* his most famous was the *Tay Bridge Disaster.* He had a strong interest in the Temperance Movement and walked to meet Queen Victoria while she was at Balmoral to read her his poetry, but was denied entry. He returned to Edinburgh in 1895, and died there penniless in 1902.

Notes

1   Johnston, *History of the Working Classes.*

2   Maureen Kerr, *George Murray. A School Teacher for St Kilda* (Islands Book Trust, 2013).

3   Quoted in Roderick Watson, *The Literature of Scotland: Middle Ages to the Nineteenth Century* (New York, N.Y: Palgrave MacMillan, 2007), p. 338.

4   'There grows a bonie brier-bush', in *The Complete Poetical Works of Robert Burns*, p. 593, ll. 1–2.

5   William Topas McGonagall, 'Brief Autobiography', in *Poetic Gems* (Dundee: David Winter and Sons, 1971), p. 68.

CHAPTER 13

Doctors and medical students

O dinna fear the doctor
He comes to mak' ye weel,
Alexander Smart

Introduction

During the 19th century, as the discoveries in medicine grew and changed clinical practice, so the doctor is described in different ways. However there are few stories which deal with the technicalities of care, most relate to personal encounters with patients. In particular the 'Kailyard' school emphasises the personal qualities of the doctor, and the importance of compassion and care. Medical students are not frequently discussed though there are a couple of important examples in the literature of Scotland in this period. The provision of a health service is an important gap in the period and is reflected in the ways in which patients are able to both obtain and pay for care.

Annals of the Parish (1821), John Galt

This is the story of a small town in the west of Scotland and covers the many issues which are described by the minister during his tenure of office. His comments on the two local medical men are perhaps relevant even now. The minister notes:

But among other improvements, I should mention that a Doctor Marigold came and settled in Cayenneville, a small round, happy tempered man, whose funny stories were far better liked than his drugs. There was doubt among the weavers, if he was a skilful Esculapian*, and this doubt led to their holding out an inducement to another medical man, Doctor Tanzy, to settle there likewise, by which it grew into a saying that Cayenneville there was a doctor for health as well as sickness. For Doctor Marigold was one of the best hands in the country at a pleasant punch bowl, while Doctor Tanzy had all the pre-requisite knowledge of the faculty for the bedside.[1]

These two important facets of medical competence remain relevant; the need for a bedside manner and clinical skills, one reason why the General Medical Council was set up in the 19th century.

Alexander Smart

Born in Montrose in 1798 Alexander Smart attended Montrose Academy. One of his teachers was 'Norval' who seemed to be a despot and was particularly fearsome in relation to corporal punishment. When punishment was due, the boys were ordered to bend over a long wooden bench, to which they were bound so that there was no escape while the master, Mr Norval, administered the requisite number of strokes of his tawse (belt) across legs and bottoms. In spite of this Smart became an apprentice watchmaker then moved to Edinburgh. He became a printer and editor and publisher of the *Montrose Chronicle,* subsequently moving to the *Dundee Courier*. He published a number of poems and then a small book called *Rambling Rhymes* which was well received. In 1845 he published an enlarged volume of poems. He was a major contributor to *Whistle-Binkie* from which this poem from the 'Songs from a Nursery' section comes. It was to be sung to the tune 'Gin a body meets a body'.

The Doctor

O dinna fear the doctor
He comes to mak' ye weel,
To nurse ye like a tender flower.
And your wee head to heal;

---

* A follower of (A) Esculapius, the Greek God of Medicine and Healing.

He brings the bloom back to your cheek,
The blythe blink to your e'e-
An't werena for the doctor
My bonnie bairn might dee.

O wha would fear the doctor!
His pouthers, pills an' a'
Ye just a wee bit swither gi'e,
An' then the taste's awa'!
He'll mak' ye sleep as sound's a tap
And rise as light's a flee-
An't werena for the doctor
My bonnie bairn might dee,

A kind man is the doctor,
As mony poor folk ken;
He spares nae toil by day or night
To ease them o' their pain;
And O he lo'es the bairnies weel,
An' taks them on his knee-
An't werena for the doctor
My bonnie bairn might dee.[2]

This poem is reflective of all the good characteristics of the doctor. Pleasant, kind, hardworking and ever anxious to help.

'Rab and his Friends', John Brown

This is a short story by Dr John Brown (1810–1882) and was introduced in the first chapter of this book. John Brown was a general practitioner in Edinburgh who wrote a series of short stories, often with a medical context. 'Rab' is a tale of a medical student in Edinburgh in the days before anaesthetics. The characters of this story were introduced in Chapter 1: Ailie the patient with breast cancer, James her husband and Rab the dog. It is narrated by the medical student. Her first discussion with the doctor was noted in my first chapter.

Ailie is taken to theatre and the process is described by a medical student:

The operating theatre is crowded; much talk and fun, and all the cordiality and stir of youth. The surgeon with his staff of assistants is there. In comes Ailie: one look at her quiets and abates the eager students. That beautiful old woman is too much for them; they sit down, and are dumb, and gaze at her. These rough boys feel the power of her presence. She walks in quickly, but without haste; dressed in her mutch, her neckerchief, her white dimity shortgown, her black bambazeen petticoat, showing her white worsted stockings and her carpet shoes. Behind her was James, with Rab. James sat down in the distance, and took that huge and noble head between his knees. Rab looked perplexed and dangerous; for ever cocking his ear and dropping it as fast.

Ailie stepped up on a seat, and laid herself on the table, as her friend the surgeon told her; arranged herself, gave a rapid look at James, shut her eyes, rested herself on me, and took my hand. The operation was at once begun; it was necessarily slow; and chloroform – one of God's best gifts to his suffering children – was then unknown. The surgeon did his work. The pale face showed its pain, but was still and silent. Rab's soul was working within him; he saw that something strange was going on , – blood flowing from his mistress, and she suffering; his ragged ear was up, and importunate; he growled and gave now and then a sharp impatient yelp; he would have liked to have done something to that man. But James had him firm, and gave him a glower from time to time, and an intimation of a possible kick; – all the better for James, it kept his eye and his mind off Ailie.

It is over: she is dressed, steps gently and decently down from the table, looks for James; then, turning to the surgeon and students, she curtsies, – and in a low, clear voice, begs their pardon if she has behaved ill. The students – all of us – wept like children; the surgeon happed her up carefully, – and, resting on James and me, Ailie went to her room, Rab following.

This is remarkably powerful and it is a story which bears re-reading both for its historical value, but also in terms of its role in relation to the management of a difficult disease. It is interesting to compare the management of breast cancer described in this instance, with the modern process. There was no ethical approval given, a dog and a relative were in theatre, explanations were limited, and the technology minimal. As might be predicted, she develops an infection and dies. Perhaps of relevance is the real emotional involvement of the students. They were moved and concerned and this raises issues in current clinical practice of the detachment of the doctor from the patient, and whether or not this is appropriate. Interestingly, in a recent book for teenagers *Fleshmarket* by Nicola Morgan[3] in which the dealings of Dr Knox of 'body snatchers' fame are described, the first chapter mirrors the story of Rab.

Dr John Brown also wrote a short story entitled 'Marjorie Fleming'.[4] This is the story of a young lady, aged nine, who clearly had precocious powers of writing, reading and conversation. She was a very close friend and confidante of Sir Walter Scott, who took her places and indeed showed her off. She died tragically at the age of nine of measles. He is devastated at the outcome and this illustrates the emotional bonds which are developed during illness. This might be between the patient, and friends and relatives, or with the clinical staff providing the care.

Another of his stories, 'Dr Francis Adams of Banchory', highlights the academic breadth of doctors.[5] Adams was a general practitioner in the small village of Banchory in Deeside near Aberdeen. He was a highly respected GP, but as he rode around his practice he had a board in front of him on which was placed the works of the Greek classics, which he translated as he travelled to visit patients. His translation of the works of Hippocrates was highly regarded and he was invited to be professor of Greek at Oxford. He declined this, preferring to visit his patients in Banchory. In this piece, *Francis Adams,* two important characteristics are set out: the first being the wish to care for patients, and the second, the breadth of interest of the doctor.

It is interesting to note that Dr John Brown was widely regarded as a writer, and the following poem by Robert Louis Stevenson, highlights both his writing and 'Rab and his Friends':

To Dr John Brown. By RLS

(Whan the dear doctor, dear to a'
Was still amang us here belaw
I set my pipes his praise to blaw
Wi' a' my speerit
But no, Dear Doctor! He's awa'
And ne'er can hear it.)

By Lyne and Tyne, by Thames and Tees'
By a' the various river-Deeds,
In Mars and Manors 'yont the sea
Or here at hame
Whaure'er there's kindly folk to please
They ken your name

They ken your name, they ken your tyke,
They ken the honey from your byke,
But mebbe after a' your fyke,
(The truth to tell)
It's just your honest Rab they like,
an' no yoursel'.

As at the gowff, some canny play
Should tee a common ba' wi' care
His souple shintie –
An the ba' rise into the air
A leevin' lintie

Saw in the games we writers play,
There comes to some a bonny day,
When a dear ferlie shall repay
Their years of strife,
An' like your Rab, their things o' clay
Spread wings o' life.[6]

The Surgeon's Daughter, Sir Walter Scott

In this novel, written in 1823, Scott sets out some of the important characteristics of the doctor and of the medical student and the role they played in
rural life. The narrator writes:

> The exquisitely beautiful portrait which the Rambler has painted of his
> friend Levett, well describes Gideon Gray and many other village doctors,
> from whom Scotland reaps more benefit, and to whom she is perhaps more
> ungrateful than to any other class of men, excepting her schoolmasters. Such
> a rural man of medicine is usually the inhabitant of some pretty borough or
> village, which forms the central part of his practice. But, besides attending
> to such cases as the village may afford, he is day and night at the service of
> everyone who may command his assistance within a circle of forty miles in
> diameter, untraversed by roads in many directions, including moors, moun-
> tains, rivers and lakes. For the dangerous journeys through an inaccessible
> country for services of the most essential kind, rendered at the expense, or
> risk at least, of his own health and life, the Scottish village doctor receives
> at best a very moderate recompense, often one which is totally inadequate,
> and very frequently none whatever. He has none of the ample resources
> proper to the brothers of the profession in an English town. The burgesses
> of a Scottish borough are rendered, by their limited means of luxury, inac-
> cessible to gout, surfeits, and all the comfortable chronic diseases, which
> are attendant on wealth and indolence. Four years or so of abstemiousness,
> enable them to stand an election dinner; and there is no hope of broken
> heads among a score or two of quiet electors, who settle the business over
> a table. There the mothers of the state never make a point of pouring, in the
> course of every revolving year, a certain quantity of doctor's stuff through
> the bowels of their beloved children. Every old woman, from the Townhead
> to the Townfit, can prescribe a dose of salts, or spread a plaster; and it is
> only when a fever or palsy renders matters serious, that the assistance of the
> doctor is invoked by his neighbours in the borough.
>
> But still the man of science cannot complain of inactivity or want of prac-
> tice. If he does not find patients at his door, he seeks them though a wide
> circle. Like the ghostly lover of Burger's Leonora, he mounts at midnight,

and traverses in the darkness, . . . when the arrives at such a stately termination of his journey, where his services are required,, either to bring a wretch into this world, or prevent one from leaving it, the scene of misery is often such, that, far from touching the hard-saved shilling which are gratefully offered to him, he bestows his medicines as well as his attendance – for charity . . . In short there is no creature in Scotland that works harder, and is more poorly requited than the country doctor, unless perhaps it may be his horse. Yet the horse is, and indeed must be, hardy, active and indefatigable, in spite of a rough coat and indifferent condition; and so you will often find in his master, under an unpromising and blunt exterior, professional skill and enthusiasm, intelligence, humanity, courage and science.

Mr Gideon Gray, surgeon in the village of Middlemas, situated in the midland counties of Scotland, led the rough, active, and ill-rewarded course of life which we have endeavoured to describe.[7]

Tom Hilary (an attorney's apprentice) says that the parson lives by the sins of the people, the lawyer by their distresses, and the doctor by their diseases.

On the morning after this gay evening, the two young meds (medical students) were labouring together in a plot of ground . . . which the Doctor had converted into a garden, where he raised, with a view to a pharmacy as well as botany, some rare plants, which obtained the place from the vulgar the sounding name of the Physic Garden.

The detail given paints an idyllic picture of the doctor and the inquisitive medical students, helping to set out the physic garden, the role of the doctor in caring and the ability to respond to the needs of patients.

Rob Roy (1817), Sir Walter Scott

This romantic novel is based mainly in the west of Scotland, but in the introduction Scott notes a link with a distinguished medical person, who is often referred to in literature of the period. Scott comments:

But while in the city of Aberdeen, Rob Roy met a relation of a different class and character from those whom he was sent to summon to arms. This was

Dr James Gregory, (by descent a MacGregor) the patriarch of a dynasty of professors distinguished for literary and scientific talent, and grandfather of the late eminent physician and accomplished scholar, Professor Gregory of Edinburgh. This gentleman was at the time Professor of Medicine in King's College Aberdeen, and son of Dr James Gregory, distinguished in science and inventor of the reflecting telescope. With such a family it may seem our friend Rob could have little in communion . . . He invited Rob Roy to his house, treated him with so much kindness, that he produced in his bosom a degree of gratitude which seemed likely to occasion very inconvenient effects.[8]

He meets Dr Gregory's son and determines to take him away from useless book learning and make a man of him. An appropriate way is found to say no! There is however a sequel:

James Gregory, who thus escaped being his kinsman's recruit, and in all probability his Henchman, was afterward professor of medicine in the College (Edinburgh), and, like most of his family distinguished by his scientific acquirements. He was rather of an irritable and pertinacious disposition; and his friends were wont to remark, when he showed any symptom of these foibles, 'Ah! This comes of not having been educated by Rob Roy'.

While in Glasgow, near the old College, there is a scene in *Rob Roy* recorded in a pharmacy: the narrator writes:

I stopped at a small unpretending shop, the sign of which intimated the indweller to be Christopher Nielson, surgeon and apothecary, I requested of the little boy who was pounding some stuff in a mortar that he would procure with me an audience with this learned pharmacopolist. He opened the door of the back-shop, where I found a lively elderly man. . .and I gave him an account of being accidentally wounded by the button breaking off my antagonist's foil. When he applied some lint and something else he thought proper to the trifling wound . . . he observed 'There never was a button on the foil that made this hurt . . . But we surgeons are a secret generation – if it werena for hot blood and ill blood, what would become of the two learned faculties?'

183

Finally, in *Rob Roy,* there is another reference to limes. 'The limes', he assured us, 'were from his own little farm yonder-awa' (indicating the West Indies with a knowing shrug of his shoulders).' This is further evidence of the important, and contemporary, link between Glasgow and the Americas for tobacco and fruit. It also relates directly to health issues and the culture in cities like Glasgow and Liverpool with their major tobacco importing and production facilities.

Treasure Island (1883), Robert Louis Stevenson

This classic adventure story is set in Bristol and moves to a mysterious Treasure Island.[9] Stevenson's father was the builder of many lighthouses, including Muckle Flugga in Unst, the most northerly lighthouse in Britain and it has been said that the map of Treasure Island was created from the map of Unst. In an article in *The Scotsman* in 1962 A.T. Cluness goes through the book, and the map, and makes a convincing case for the comparison.[10]

There is an additional dimension to this. In the *Times Literary Supplement* (TLS) of 18th November, 2011, there was an article by John Sutherland, 'Stories for Boys' which relates to the writing of *Treasure Island*.[11] In the summer months of 1881, Stevenson with his wife Fanny Osbourne and her son Lloyd went to Braemar on Deeside in the Scottish Highlands to improve his health. The weather was terrible and they read for a few days. Lloyd spent his time drawing, and at one point Stevenson joined him and drew a map, that of 'Treasure Island.' Thereafter he wrote a chapter of the book every morning and read it to the family at lunch. The following week in the TLS there was a letter from L.A. Yeats whose relative lived close to Stevenson's cottage, and they became friends. His relative's name was John Silver, perhaps a coincidence.[12]

The tale begins in the Admiral Benbow Inn, and early on we are introduced to the serious and stable character of Dr Livesey, a medical doctor and magistrate. At the start he shows his clinical skill. The Captain has just called for rum, then falls to the ground. Dr Livesey pops in and is asked to help. The crew shout:

'Oh doctor', we cried, 'What shall we do? Where is he wounded?'

'Wounded? A fiddle stick's end' said the doctor. 'No more wounded then you or I'

He then proceeds with the help of Jim, the young hero of the novel, to bleed him to prevent a stroke. This points to a link between high alcohol consumption and the risk of stroke.

The Captain recovers and has fine words for the doctor when he asks Jim to bring him more rum. Jim protests and the Captain replies in the following manner:

'Doctors is all swabs', he says, 'and that doctor there, what do he know about seafaring me? I've been in places as hot as pitch, and mates dropping round with Yellow Jack [yellow fever] and the blessed land a-heaving like the sea with earthquakes – what do the doctor know of lands like that? And I lived on rum, I tell you.'

Dr Livesey gets involved in the preparation for the journey, but to continue, he has to get a physician from London to take charge of his practice while he was away. Locums were difficult to get even then.

Another medical event is the recollection of Long John Silver's amputation and his wooden leg. 'It was a master surgeon, him that ampytated me – out of college and all – Latin by the bucket and what not; but he was hanged like a dog, and sun-dried like the rest, at Corso Castle.'

Near the end of the book the pirates have returned home, but are on parole in a block-house and Dr Livesey is asked to visit them. He meets Jim and the pirates, and then says

'Well, Well . . . duty first and pleasure later.' A moment later he had entered the block-house, and, with one grim nod to me, proceeded with his work among the sick. He seemed under no apprehension, though he must have known that his life, among these treacherous demons, depended on a hair; and he rattled on to his patients as if he were paying an ordinary professional visit in a quiet English family. His manner, I suppose reacted on the men; for they behaved to him as if nothing had occurred – as if he were still ship's doctor and they still faithful friends before the mast.

He asks them how they are, and if they have taken their medicines, and rebukes them for camping in a bog on the island, and that they might now have malaria.

The picture of the doctor, doing his work as a professional, interacting with the men being an important aspect of that work and reflects perhaps on the doctors who treated Stevenson over many years and whose help is recorded in *Underwoods*.

Underwoods (1887), Robert Louis Stevenson

This is a collection of poems in Scots and English and begins with a remarkable dedication to doctors, as I noted in my first chapter. Stevenson also notes:

> Gratitude is but a lame sentiment; thanks, when they are expressed, are often more embarrassing than welcome; and yet I must set forth mine to a few out of many doctors who have brought me comfort and help: to Dr Willey of San Francisco, whose kindness to a stranger it must be as grateful to him, as it is touching to me, to remember; to Dr Karl Ruedi of Davos, the good genius of the English in his frosty mountains; to Dr Herbert of Paris, whom I knew only for a week, and to Dr Caissot of Montpellier, whom I knew only for ten days, and who have written their names deeply in my memory; to Dr Brandt of Royat; to Dr Wakefield of Nice; to Dr Chepmell, whose visits make it a pleasure to be ill; to Dr Horace Dobell, so wise in counsel; to Sir Andrew Clark, so unwearied in kindness and to that wise youth, my uncle, Dr Balfour.

> I forget as many as I remember; and I ask both to pardon me, these for silence, those for inadequate speech. But one name I have kept on purpose to the last, because it is a household word with me, and because if I had not received favours from so many hands and in so many quarters of the world, it should have stood upon this page alone; that of my friend Thomas Bodley Scott of Bournemouth. Will he accept this, although shared among so many, for a dedication to himself? And when next my ill-fortune (which has thus its pleasant side) brings him hurrying to me when he would fain sit down to meat or lie down to rest, will he care to remember that he takes this trouble for one who is not fool enough to be ungrateful? RLS

Stevenson pays tribute to a number of doctors across the world who have helped him during his illnesses. Stevenson always had a 'weak chest' and this has always been considered to be tuberculosis. However there are some suggestions that it could have been bronchiectasis, or even sarcoidosis. It is relevant to pick out two of the doctors named for further discussion.

Stevenson specifically sets apart Thomas Bodley Scott for special mention. In his obituary in the *British Medical Journal* 16th February 1924, Scott's career is set out.[13] He was born in Brighton, and a direct descendant of Sir Thomas Bodley who founded the Bodleian Library in Oxford. Educated at St Bartholomew's Hospital he moved to Bournemouth where he established himself in general practice. He was a man of great charm and endowed with exceptional tact and commonsense. He looked after Stevenson when he stayed in Bournemouth. Stevenson wrote that he had been of great help to him. Dr Scott used to recall how Stevenson said to him one morning. 'I've got a shilling shocker' and then narrated to him a dream he had had, which formed the basis of *Dr Jekyll and Mr Hyde*. Dr Scott was one of those who persuaded Stevenson to make his home abroad.

In addition he mentions Sir Andrew Clark who was born in Aberdeen and had his medical education there and in Edinburgh. He worked in pathology with Dr John Hughes Bennett and was assistant demonstrator to Robert Knox, of 'body snatcher's' fame. He moved to London and established a very large and fashionable practice. Interestingly he wrote numerous books and had a particular interest in lung diseases.

Such was the quality of medical advice Stevenson received during his many episodes of illness.

Beside the Bonnie Brier Bush (1895), Ian Maclaren[14]

> There grows a bonnie brier bush in our kail-yard,
> And white are the blossoms on't in our kail-yard.[15]

Maclaren set the tone for many of the Kailyard writings, and the coinage of the term 'Kailyard' comes from the poem whose first line is used as the title of this novel.

The first section considers 'Domsie' the familiar name for the dominie, the local school teacher in the village of Drumtochty. 'Drumtochty was a name in thae days wi' the lads he sent tae college'. The dialogue is all male, no women were sent to college. The dominie is aided by the doctor and the local minister. He was a great scholar and a credit to the parish.

'He had an unerring scent for a lad o' pairts [a promising boy] in "his laddies"'. He could detect a scholar in the egg and prophesised Latinity from a boy that seemed fit only to be a cowherd. Dromtochty always had a student at the university.

Seven ministers, four schoolmasters, four doctors, one professor and three civil service men had been sent out by the auld schule in Domsie's time, besides many that had given themselves to mercantile purposes.

There was just a single ambition in those humble homes, to have one of its members at college and if Domsie approved a lad, then his brothers and sisters would give their wages, and the family would live on skimmed milk and oat cake to let him have his chance.

It was awfu work the next twa years, but the Doctor stood in weel with the Greek. Ye mind how Geordie tramped ower the muir to the manse and thro' the weet an' snaw, and there was aye dry stockings for him in the kitchen afore he had his Greek in the Doctor's study.

And a warm drink tae,' put in Margaret, 'and that's the window I pit a light in to guide him hame in the dark winter nights.

George goes off to college and there is anticipation about the outcome; will he, or will he not get a prize? At last the letter arrived. 'Dear Mr Jamieson, the class honour lists are out, and you will be pleased to know that I have got the medal both in the Humanity and the Greek.'

Telling his mother was another task:

Margaret met us at the end of the house beside the brier bush, where George was to sit on summer afternoons before he died. 'Under God, this was your doings Maister Jamieson, and for your reward ye'ill get neither silver or gold, but ye hae a mither's gratitude.'

George eventually comes home and Margaret watches from the window and sees his face. It told her plain what she had feared. 'When their eyes met and before she helped him down, mother and son understood.' His mother notes: 'When I found George wrapped in his plaid beside the brier bush whose roses were no whiter than his cheeks' she understands what has happened, he is ill, and the whiteness and tiredness suggest tuberculosis. He gives away his favourite books, and there is a Christian justification for his illness. Finally there is the funeral of the scholar attended by his college friends. They were 'each of his own type, and could only have met in the commonwealth of letters', one from an ancient Scottish House, high church and Tory, the other from a fishing croft in Barra.

Following the funeral there is a confession from one of the students. Geordie helped him through even when his disease was heavy upon him. His white face was shining and 'He pulled me oot of hell'.

This is a remarkable story which was replicated across Scotland; the teacher recognising the bright boy, the community helping and ultimate success. The story ends in tragedy with the death of the young man from a now preventable and treatable disease. The comment on the value of the university and the 'commonwealth of letters' is also fascinating, and an indication of the value placed on places of learning.

A Doctor of the Old School (1895), Ian McLaren[16]

This is the quintessential 'good doctor' story. The preface sets out the context and is written for an American audience. McLaren has two things to say to his readers:

> One is to answer a question that has been often and fairly asked. Was there ever any doctor so self-forgetful and so utterly Christian as William MacLure? To which I am proud to reply, on my conscience: Not one man, but many in Scotland and in the South country. I will dare prophecy also across the sea.
>
> It has been one man's good fortune to know four country doctors, not

one of whom was without his faults-Weelun was not perfect-but who, each one, might have sat for my hero.

Then I desire to thanks my readers, chiefly the medical profession for the reception given to the Doctor of Drumtochty.

Then follows an introduction, the village and the people, their clothes and dietary habits, and the weather have a significant influence. The cold and wet produce a 'hoast' or cough, and the women folk ask the head of the house to 'Change his feet' if he had walked through a burn on his way home. The narrator notes:

> When illness had the audacity to attack a Drumtochty man, it was described as a 'whup', and treated by the men with a fine negligence. Hillocks was sitting in the Post Office one afternoon when I looked in for my letters, and the right side of his face was blazing red. His subject of discourse was the prospects of the turnip 'breer', but he casually explained that he was waiting for the doctor . . . . The doctor made his diagnosis from horseback on sight, and stated the result with that admirable clearness which endeared him to Drumtochty.

With people with little money and of such poor health, the doctor has to cover neighbouring parishes to earn a living. The Drumtochty postman carried word if the doctor was needed, and the doctor 'did his best for the need of every man, woman and child in this wild, straggling district, year in, year out, in the snow, in the heat, in the dark and in the light, without rest, and without holidays for forty years.' As indeed his father before him had done, though he disliked being called out for something trivial. 'But he's no veera ceevil gin ye bring him when there's naethin' wrang.' His treatment was fairly limited. When called to a patient with 'naethin' wrang' he comments 'Gie him a gude dose o' castor oil and stop his meat for a day, an' he'll be a' richt in the morn'. For all this his fees were pretty much what the people chose to give him and the collected then once a year at the Kildrummie fair.

Much was expected of him. For example he goes to see Annie, the wife of Tammas, who is seriously ill. He is distraught and makes the point 'A' wer'na prepared for this, for a' aye thocht she wude live langest.' The doctor tries to comfort Tammas, and Tammas replies with a question:

'Can naethin' be dune, doctor? Ye savit Flora Cammil, and young Burnbrae, and yon shepherd's wife Dunleith wy, an' we were a sae prood o' ye, an' pleased tae think that ye hed keepit deith frae anither hame. Can ye no think o' somethin' tae help Annie, and gie her back tae her man and bairns?'

And the doctor replies in turn:

'Tammas my poor fellow, if it could avail, a' tell ye a' wud lay doon this auld worn-oot ruckle o'a body of mine just tae see ye baith sittin' at the fireside, an' the bairns roon ye, couthy and cantie again; but it's no tae be Tammas, it's no tae be.'

Then the doctor goes to see an old friend, who says that there might be a specialist who could treat her but it would cost 100 guineas, such a huge sum, but he says he will pay, and they send a telegraph to Edinburgh for Sir George. He arrives by train the next day and is met on the platform by the doctor. It is an eventful journey to get to see Annie over fields and through streams, and they had difficulty in keeping the surgical instruments out of the water. The surgeon operates in the barn, as the dog outside barks. The operation is over and the patient saved. A cheque is given to Sir George, but he refuses it. As the train leaves the station Sir George reminds the doctor to mind the antiseptic dressings. Even the knighted surgeon has high moral principles.

Infection was another problem. There is another story, 'A fight with death' where a London doctor, visiting a local shooting lodge, says that Saunders has caught the infection on an adventurous visit to Glasgow, and gives him six hours to live. However he has not considered the role of Dr MacLure and the constitution of Saunders. There is the contrast between the country life with the soft life in the big city. Dr MacLure declares:

'Ye see, when onybody gets as low as puir Saunders here, its just a hand to hand wrestle atween the fever and his constitution, an' of course if he had been a shilpit, stuntit, fechless effeegy o' a cratur, fed on tea an' made dishes and pushioned wi' bad air, Saunders wud hae nae chance; he wes boond tae gae out like the snuff o' a candle.

191

But Sauders has been fillin' his lungs for five and thirty years wi' strong Dromtochty air, and eating naethin' but kirny aitmeal, and drinking naethin' but fresh milk frae the coo, an' followin' the ploo through the new turned sweet smellin' earth, an'swinging the scythe in haytime and harvest, till the legs an' airms o' him were iron, and his chest wes like the cuttin' o' and oak tree.'

There is little resource available to help. MacLure makes the point

'The doctors in the toons hae nurses an' o' kinds o' handy apparatus. But you and me 'ill need tae be nurse the nicht, an' use sic things as we hev.

'There's twa dangers ahead-that Saunders' strength fails, an' that the force of the fever grows; and we have just two weapons. Yon milk on the drawers' head and a bottle of whisky is to keep up the strength, and this cool caller water is tae keep doon the fever.'

Eventually Saunders recovers, and everyone is happy, and the doctor attempts the Highland Fling in his delight. There are prayers to be said and thanks to the doctor.

The final story concerns the doctor's last journey. He is getting older, his hair is turning grey, and Annie Mitchell has knitted a huge comforter for him. Hillocks intercepts him with hot drinks, Flora Campbell brings a wonderful compound of honey and whisky for his cough and his cupboard is filled with black jam as a healing measure. The doctor gradually realises what is going on – his patients are looking after him. In the cold winter he weakens, and can hardly get out of bed. They hang a plaid over the window to break the power of the wind. He talks about the things that have happened over the years, and of his wish to do his best. His house has little furniture and no possessions, and he 'dinna keep buiks' and did not charge much of the time. And his advice to his old friend, 'If onybody need a doctor an' canna pay for him, see he's no left tae dee when a'm oot o' the road.' He knows his time has come and the parish needs a younger man'. He has left all the money he has to help others.

He confesses, 'A' did what a' cud tae keep up wi' the new medicine, but a' hed little time for readin' and nane for traivellin'. A'm the last of the auld schule.' He asks his old friend to put up a prayer, which he does with many pauses. Then he says his mother's prayer which he has done every night of his life:

> This night I lay me done to sleep
> I pray the Lord my soul to keep
> And if I die before I wake
> I pray the Lord my soul to take.

He is sleeping quietly and imagines that word had come that someone needed him. He becomes delirious and dies with a look of peace on his face, as someone who has rested from his labours.

Not surprisingly the mourning in the glen is substantial, and people come from far and wide to the funeral, all with their stories of the doctor and his kindness.

This is a remarkable story, which illustrates how far we have come, not only in terms of treatment options, but in the provision of health services. The doctor now needs to keep up to date and be regularly re-accredited.

The Little Minister, J.M. Barrie[17]

> The life of everyman is a diary in which he means to write one story, writes another; and his humblest hour is when he compares the volume as it is with what he vowed to make it.

Gavin Dishart has been groomed for the ministry. At twelve he goes to the university, and gets home at night though money is tight. He is an Auld Licht minister (traditional). His mother Margaret usually has a supper of potatoes and dripping ready.

Dr McQueen is the local doctor:

> . . . For Thrums folk seldom called in a doctor until it was too late to cure them, and Dr McQueen was not the man to pay social visits. Of skills we knew fearsome stories, as that, by looking at Archie Allardyce, who had come to broken bones on a ladder, he discovered which rung Archie fell

from. When he entered a stuffy room he would poke his staff through the window to let in fresh air then fling down a shilling for the breakage. He was deaf in the right ear, and therefore usually took the left side of prosy people, thus, as he explained, making a blessing of an affliction. 'A pity I don't hear better?'

A key scene in the book is the visit of McQueen and Gavin to Nanny Webster who lives in a mud house. She has no money and is to be sent to the poor-house. It is a tragic scene: no friends, no possessions, no hope. Humiliated she does not want the neighbours to see her. When they have come to take her away they emphasise how nice the poorhouse will be and that it will be possible to visit her. She doesn't want anyone to visit her and see her face again, and will not come out except in a hearse. As it turns out she is saved at the last minute by Babbie 'the Egyptian' (the gypsy). She needs just seven shillings a week to live on.

Gavin is at one point invited in to Dr McQueen's Surgery. Gavin comments:

It was to the doctor the cosiest room in the house, but to me and many others it was a room that smelled of hearses. On top of the pipes and tobacco tins that littered the table there usually lay a death certificate, placed there deliberately by the doctor to scare his sister, who had a passion for putting the surgery to rights.

'By the way,' McQueen said, after he and Gavin had talked a little while, 'did I ever advise you to smoke?' 'It is your usual form of salutation' Gavin answered, laughing. 'But I don't think you ever supplied me with a reason' 'I dare say not. I am too experienced a doctor to cheapen my prescriptions in that way. However, here is one good reason. I have noticed sir, that at your age, a man is either slave to a pipe, or to a woman. Do you want me to lend you a pipe now?'

Not the best justification for taking tobacco.

Later in the story the Minister notes,

'Vaguely I knew that Nanny had put the kettle on the fire – a woman's first thought when there is illness in the house.'

'Dr McQueen was Gavin's best man. He died long ago of scarlet fever. So severe was the epidemic that for a week he was never in bed. He attended fifty cases without suffering, but as soon as he bent over Hendry Munn's youngest boys, who both had it, he said "I'm smitted", and went home to die.'

These stories are emotional and sentimental, but struck a chord with the public and the books were widely distributed. They help to create the image of the devoted doctor, with no interest in money, only for the care of his patients. Even William McGonagall has a good word for his doctor. McGonagall writes:

A tribute to Dr Murison, William McGonagall.

Success to the good and skilful Dr Murison,
The golden opinions he has won
From his patients one and all,
And from myself, McGonagall.

He is very skilful and void of pride;
He was so to me when at my bedside,
When I turned badly on the 25th of July,
And was ill with inflammation, and like to die.

A tribute indeed from the poetic master![18]

Galoshins. The Scottish Folk Play [19]

The context

The Galoshins is a folk play performed in the central belt of Scotland, Angus, the Borders, and Dumfries and Galloway. It was performed continuously in Biggar from mediaeval times and its heyday was in the middle of the 19th century. It was transmitted by oral tradition and by chapbooks. In Glasgow it could be bought at a bookshop called 'The Poet's Box.'

It was generally performed around the turn of the year. Troops of children attended and were given gifts of sweets, fruit, plum cake, and money. Funding it was a problem for the performance as it was akin to begging and the tradition gradually fell away, especially after World War II. Its relevance here is that the doctor is the main character and is retained in all performances throughout the period and venues.

The performance

The play was performed in theatrical style, the doctor being in top hat and evening dress or morning dress. Guising – the assumption of another identity by the use of a costume – was part of the process and as was disguising – the concealment of personal identity. The name of the knight in the story could be Alexander, Caesar, Bruce or Wallace. The key feature was that the doctor had a cure.

Galloshins is a death and resurrection drama and is known only in Scotland. The words were not recorded in writing until early 19th century. The name could be related to galloche – wooden shoes, and scholars in universities admitted of no college but lying in the town . . . commonly wear galloches.

The play

There are many versions of the play, depending on where it was performed. The titles indicate the place in Scotland from where each version originated. Here are a few from the Abbotsford version:

Abbotsford

Here comes in a doctor
The best that Scotland ever produced
I have gone from nation to nation to learn my trade
And now I've come back to Scotland to cure the dead

I can cure the pox and the blue devils
The rumelgumption in an old man's belly
The rumplel-grane and the Brandy-whirtelz

And can raise the man fresh and hale
That had lain seven year in his grave

Yes I have a bottle here that
Hangs by my side they call it Hoxy Croxy
Now I'll put it to his nose
And a little to his bum and say
Jack rises up and fight again and it is done.

Now once I was dead
But now I am alive
An blessed are the hands of those
That made me to revive.

What can you cure
The clap and the gangrene
And an old man in his grave
Seven years and twenty more

Each of the versions has a slightly different variation on the theme, this one is from Stirling:

Once I was deid, sir, noo I am alive;
Blessed be the doctor that made me revive!
We'll a' join hands and never fight more,
We'll a' be guid brithers, as we hae been afore.

There are fascinating references to illness and to the way in which the doctor had learned his trade, often in countries abroad. In each, however, is the expectation that the doctor would cure the patient, and all would be well. He does this with a bottle, the contents of which are unclear, but it does the job. He may also carry a wand, a rod, a bundle of herbs or a club, all of which have the same powers.

Mona Maclean, Margaret Todd – Women in medicine

One interesting example of life as a medical student is that of Mona Maclean, which tells the story of women in medicine. A novel, *Mona Maclean* was written in 1892 by Margaret Todd, a medical student and doctor associated with Sophia Jex-Blake and other women in the late 1900s studying medicine.[20] Its subtitle is *Medical Student* and is written under the pseudonym Graham Travers. It begins in London as the results of the Intermediate MB (Bachelor of Medicine) results are posted, and Mona, a student at University College, has failed again. The scene is typical with crowds of students trying to see who has passed and failed. She is devastated and returns to Scotland, and the family, where she spends several months thinking about what to do. She inevitably meets a young man who is also studying medicine but she does not reveal to him her own interest. This part of the story has references to vivisection, dissection and botany. There are comments on the role of women, as in this dialogue between Doris, a friend of Mona, and an elderly gentleman:

'Women' was the reply, delivered with a courteous bow, 'have no power, they have only influence.'

Doris flushed, and then said serenely, 'We won't dispute it. Influence is in the soul, of which power is the outward form.'

And again in a dialogue between two students:

'And as a natural consequence, the supply of medical women will exceed the demand in the next ten years in this country. After that, things will level themselves, I suppose; but at present, if a woman is to succeed, she must be better than the average man.'

'Whereas at present we are getting mainly the average women, and of course the average woman is inferior to the average man.'

'Heretic!'

Here is also a clear statement of why Mona (and presumably Margaret Todd) wanted to study medicine:

When Mona began her medical career she was actuated partly by intense love of study and scientific work, and partly by a firm and enthusiastic conviction that, while the fitness of women for certain spheres of usefulness is an open question, medical work is the natural right and duty of the sex, apart from all shifting standards and conventional views.

She also gives another reason for studying medicine,

'It is perfectly awful to think how helpless people are who are quite outside of the profession. I think it is worthwhile studying medicine, if only to be able to tell your friends whom to consult – or rather, whom not to consult.'

What a good reason to wish to become a doctor.

She of course returns to London and is greeted by the younger medical students as something of a hero. She helps then with anatomy and their dissections, and there are some interesting conversations between them. She sets out some of her other beliefs.

'It is pleasant is it not, to leave dusty museums now and then and feel Science growing all around one? And what I love about the University of London is that it allows for that kind of thing in its Honours papers.'

She of course passes on the next occasion and gets a first in Physiology: 'Mona Maclean, London School of Medicine for Women. Exhibition and Gold Medal.' She eventually marries her admirer, and now both doctors they set up practice together. They do not set up practice in Harley Street as advised as they 'were far too enthusiastic to forego the early days of night work, and of practice amongst the poor.' The book ends with a scene which demonstrates the essence of needing women doctors. Ralph, her husband sees a young girl as a patient. As she enters his consulting room she bursts into tears. He looks at her carefully and says,

'I think' he said kindly 'you would rather see the doctor who shares my practice.' And he rose and opened the door. Mona looked up smiling. 'Mona, dear' he said quietly, 'here is a case for you.'

Patient choice and patient needs are both satisfied. This is a quiet defence of women in medicine, and establishes their role, not just as competent, and caring doctors, but as leaders and innovators. At the start of the 21st century over 60% of entrants to medical schools in the UK are female, and they have added hugely to the profession on medicine. Mona Maclean is a break-through book and establishes that women are more than equal to men in medicine.

We have come a long way from Marion Gilchrist who graduated in Glasgow in 1894, the first woman medical graduate in Scotland.

'Seeking the Houdie', James Hogg (1770–1835)[21]

This short story by James Hogg illustrates three important aspects of health care. The first is the importance of the professional staff, in this case the houdie (sometimes spelled 'howdie') or midwife, and how the role has changed over the years. The narrator sets this out in the first paragraph of the story:

> There was a shepherd on the lands of Meggat-dale who once set out riding with might and main, under the cloud of night, for that most important and necessary personage in a remote and mountainous country, called by a different name in every country of the world, excepting perhaps Egypt and England; but by the Highlanders most expressly termed bean-glhuine, or te the toctor.

Such people, almost all women, were invaluable at a time of poor travel and communication. Which leads to the second important point, that of the provision of a health service. Robin, the horse rider, had an incredibly difficult journey seeking the houdie over fields and hills with a rather suborn horse. He was thrown and tumbles and had at times to pull the horse along. There was no NHS 24 or ambulance, just a wilful horse in the night and awkward terrain.

The third issue is the folk traditions associated with houdies, and the supernatural links which seem to occur. Robin doesn't know where he is and where he is going, and begins to call out, when an elderly woman appears dressed in coarse country garb. She kneels down and picks up something that looks like a baby. He is concerned and he asks who she is. She replies that 'it is a queer thing that a father does not recognise his ain daughter.' She also says that when they meet again he will be preparing for another world. She says his daughter has been born. He does not understand so invites her to come back with him. He tries to catch her but in the struggle she disappears. It turns out, though they cannot find her, that her name is that of Robin's new daughter. A few days before his death he sees her again. Hogg's final comments are interesting.

> Many are the traditions remaining in the country, relative to the seeking of midwives, or houdies, as they are universally denominated all over the south of Scotland; and strange adventures are related as having happened in these precipitate excursions, which were proverbially certain to happen at night. Indeed it would appear, that there hardly ever was a midwife brought, but some incident occurred indicative of the fate or fortunes of the little forthcoming stranger; but, amongst them all, I have selected this as the most remarkable.
>
> I am exceedingly grieved at the discontinuance of midwifery, that primitive and original calling, in this primitive and original country; for never were such merry groups in Scotland as the midwives and their kimmers in former days, and never was there such a store of capital stories and gossip circulated as on these occasions. But those days are over! And alack, and woe is me! No future old shepherd shall tell another tale of SEEKING THE HOUDIE!

This latter reference, and an important one of terms of medical developments, is to the rise of the 'male midwife' as the science and physiology of birthing progressed. William Smellie (1697–1763) was born in Lanark and studied medicine in Glasgow before going to London via Paris. He became the leading obstetrician and wrote a *Treatise on Midwifery* in 1752. This significantly changed practice. At the same time in London William Hunter (1718–1783), another Glasgow student who practised with William Cullen in Hamilton, had also contributed significantly and Hunter produced a beautifully illustrated book on *The Gravid Uterus,* which was a major step forward. These changes, together with the introduction of anaesthesia in labour by Sir James Young Simpson, professor of Midwifery in Edinburgh, using chloroform in 1847, changed practice even further. There was little scope for the amateur midwife until the nursing profession developed, became fully trained and expert midwives became a strong professional group. Now at the start of the 21st century the process has been reversed, and midwives are an invaluable part of the health care professions though whether they still bring a store of such 'capital stories and gossip' is not clear.

Conclusions

These extracts represent a particular view of the doctor in 19th century Scotland. They are respected, trusted and looked upon to help. They are caring, compassionate, act as advocates, and spend time with their patients. They get involved with their patients and want to do the best for them. Most of the extracts represent doctors as male, but by the end of the century there is the emergence of women in this profession. Doctors are not particularly interested in money and growing rich and some at least (e.g. Francis Adams in Banchory) have much wider interests.

It could be argued that this is simply a sentimental view of the doctor, not really based on evidence. However in historical terms from the way in which the public wanted to attend a doctor there is real evidence that the general picture is correct. There is however one major proviso.

During the early part of the century medical interventions were limited, and care and compassion might be all that could be expected. However by the end of the 19th century there was much more that could be done. Even 'Weelum' McLure recognises this as he is dying, in that he has not kept up to date and hasn't read any books. This was one of the reasons for the Medical Act of 1858 and the establishment of the General Medical Council to regulate the practice of doctors; the public needed to be reassured that the doctor was competent, and was up to date. In the 21st century this is now associated with a programme of re-accreditation. However, the role model served well, and individuals and the community benefitted from such doctors. Above all the lack of a national health service becomes obvious. With no ready way to reach clinical help – from doctors, nurses, midwives, or any of the other health professionals – the care provided, had to be limited. Add to that the need to pay for each consultation meant that even to seek advice would be restricted. This is an important lesson from this study and one which will be referred to again in subsequent chapters.

Notes

1   Galt, *Annals*, p. 134.

2   *Whistle-Binkie: A collection of songs for the social circle* (Glasgow: David Robertson, 1846). From the section on Songs for the Nursery p. 20–1.

3   Nicola Morgan, *Fleshmarket,* (London: Hodder Children's Books, 2003) pp. 3–12.

4   John Brown, 'Marjorie Fleming', *Horae Subsecivae: Third Series* (London: Adam and Charles Black, 1897), pp. 199–236.

5   John Brown, 'Dr Francis Adams of Banchory', *Horae Subsecivae: First Series* (London: Adam and Charles Black, 1897), pp. 265–75.

6   Stevenson, *Underwoods and Ballads*, pp. 73–6.

7   Walter Scott, *The Surgeon's Daughter* (London: The Caxton Publishing Company, 1903), pp. 1–2.

8   Walter Scott, *Rob Roy* (Oxford: Oxford World Classics, 2008), p. 26.

9   Robert Louis Stevenson, *Treasure Island* (London: Cassell and Company, 1950).

10 A.T. Cluness, *The Scotsman*, 1962, from a typed transcript.

11 John Sutherland, 'Stories for Boys', *Times Literary Supplement*, 18 November 2011, pp. 14–15.

12 L.A. Yeats, Letter, *Times Literary Supplement*, 25 November 2011, p. 6.

13 Obituary of Thomas Bodley Scott, *British Medical Journal*, 1 (1924), 297–8.

14 Ian Maclaren, *Beside the Bonnie Brier Bush* (New York: Dodd, Mead and Co., 1895).

15 Ibid, Frontispiece

16 Ian Maclaren, *A Doctor of the Old School* (La Vergne, TN: Kessinger Publishing, 2009).

17 J.M. Barrie, *The Little Minister* (London: Cassell and Co., 1893).

18 William McGonagall, *Last Poetic Gems* (Dundee: David Winter and Sons, 1971), p. 121.

19 Brian Hayward, ed., *Galoshins: The Scottish Folk Play* (Edinburgh: Edinburgh University Press, 1992).

20 Margaret Todd, *Mona Maclean, Medical Student* (London and Glasgow: Collins Clear Type Press, 1892).

21 James Hogg, 'Seeking the Houdie', in *The Devil and the Giro: Two Centuries of Scottish Stories* (Edinburgh: Canongate, 1989), pp. 402–411.

CHAPTER 14

Health, illness and remedies

Nothing particularly happened to me; but the small-pox came in among the weans of the parish, and the smashing (devastation) that it made of the poor bits o'bairns was indeed woeful.'

. . . about the end of November, and the measles coming in at that time in the parish, there was such a smattery of the poor weans, as had not been known for an age.' Three dead children in the clachan, and they ran out of grave diggers.

Annals of the Parish, John Galt[1]

Introduction

There are numerous publications setting out the main clinical and public health problems in the 19th century, the most important of which was infection: cholera, smallpox, measles, diphtheria and tuberculosis.[2] Injury was another major factor which impacted on health. It is interesting to note that heart disease, other than rheumatic heart disease, had a low incidence, as did cancer. Both childhood and maternal mortality were high, and malnutrition, including rickets, was common in the major cities. This had important consequences for childbearing in that rickets could distort the pelvis making delivery difficult. In addition it will be relevant to note the treatments which were available, in the light of developments in medicine during the century, and in particular any comments on anaesthesia and antisepsis. The question to be addressed is whether the literature of the period accurately reflected the incidence of disease and the clinical practice. This chapter covers the following main themes; infection, healing wells and remedies, reflections on illness and dying, and disorders of the mind. Inevitably there is some overlap between these categories.

Infection

Annals of the Parish (1821), John Galt

In the *Annals of the Parish* Galt presents a series of stories in the life of the minister, the Rev Micah Balwhidder, and the parish of Dalmailing. It covers domestic affairs and the ways in which people lived their lives. There are interesting links to external affairs, but there is little travel and newspapers are a rarity in the beginning. It is a self-contained community, though, through the course of the book, habits change and life becomes more complex. As the stories progress the impact of the wider world becomes obvious as the process of globalisation begins. In terms of health it provides a view of early 19th-century Scotland, work patterns, social life and eating habits.

The minister has been educated in the Orthodox University of Glasgow and his erudition shows in his journal entries. He makes the interesting comment, in the year 1761, on the education of women in the parish, in that the sewing women and the ladies could read and speak French better than any professor in the College of Glasgow. He notes Nanse Banks the schoolmistress had been ill but 'laying the foundation for many a worthy wife and mother.' Women's education was clearly important, but for a particular purpose.

There are fascinating glimpses of the social system. Tea drinking becomes 'very rife' and women drink it behind the hedges so as not to be seen. The minister makes the comment:

> . . . and no doubt it had been laced with conek [cognac] for they were all cracking like pen-guns. But I gave them a sign by a loud host [cough] … for I heard them guilty creatures, whispering and gathering up their truck pots, and trenchers, and cowering away home.

Health issues are regularly noted. For example Balwhidder comments:

> Nothing particularly happened to me; but the small-pox came in among the weans of the parish, and the smashing (devastation) that it made of the poor bits o'bairns was indeed woeful.' He also notes in 1774, '. . . my son Gilbert was seized with the smallpox, about the beginning of December, and was

blinded by them for seventeen days; for the inoculation was not in practice yet among us, saving only in the genteel families, that went into Edinburgh for the education of their children, where it was performed by the faculty there.

Smallpox and vaccination is a recurring theme.

He records a rather difficult problem. Nanse Birrel, a distiller of herbs and well versed in the healing of sores, and who had a great following among the quarriers and colliers, 'she having gone to the physic well in the sandy hills to draw water, was found with her feet uppermost in the well . . .'

The minister's eldest son is born safely and his wife has no problems with 'the down-lying'. The howdie (midwife) says she had an easy time of it. He has a problem himself though:

> . . . I walked to the yett without my hat, by which I took a sore cold in my head, that brought on a dreadful toothache; insomuch, that I was obliged to go into Irville (Irvine) to get my tooth drawn, and this caused my face to swell to such a fright that, on the Sabbath day I could not preach to my people.

Contact with the world increases and he notes the relevance of the newspaper:

> A wonderful interest was raised amongst us all to hear of what was going on in the world, insomuch that I myself was no longer contented with the relation of news of the month in the Scots Magazine, but joined with my father-in-law Mr Kibbock, to get a newspaper twice a week from Edinburgh. As for Lady Macadam, being naturally an impatient woman, she had one sent to her three times week from London, so we had something fresh five times very week; and the old papers were sent out to families who had friends in the wars.

Reference is also made to taking a daily London newspaper for the spinners and weavers, who paid a penny a week for the same. The weavers were a trade renowned for their learning and reading capacity. They also had the ability to get any book they wished from London. His own daughter is also mentioned in this regard. The minister notes:

> . . . the coming home of my daughter Janet from the Ayr boarding school where she had learnt to play the spinet, and was becoming a conversible lassie, with a competent knowledge, for a woman, of geography and history.

By 1802 'not only was there a handsome bookseller's shop in Cayenneville, with London newspapers daily, but magazines and reviews and other publications'.

Other health incidents are noted. Lady Macadam, for example:

> . . . was stricken with the paralytics and her face was so thrown in the course of a few minutes . . . A doctor was gotten by all speed by an express, but her ladyship was smitten beyond the reach of medicine.

Infection remained a significant problem, and he describes a typical episode; '. . . about the end of November, and the measles coming in at that time in the parish, there was such a smattery of the poor weans, as had not been known for an age.' Three dead children in the clachan, and they ran out of grave diggers. He notes the role of the doctor in these circumstances, 'death is the grim creditor, and a doctor but brittle bail (temporary release) when the hour of reckoning is at hand.'

Death is always present and Balwhidder notes:

> In the month of February my second wife was gathered to the Lord. She had been ill for some time with an income [pain] in her side, which no medicine could remove. I had the best doctors in the countryside to her, but their skill was of no avail, their opinions being that her ail was caused by an internal abscess, for which physic has provided no cure.

Shortly after his wife dies he comments 'I saw that it would be necessary, as soon as decency would allow for me to have another wife. This to look after the servant lassies, look after the money and the house.' As a result he looks for a widow or an older single woman.

The Surgeon's Daughter, Sir Walter Scott

This book describes the lives of people in a small rural borough. Smallpox arrives:

> While the parents were in this agony of apprehension, the General's principal servant, a native of Northumberland like himself, informed him one morning that there was a young man from the same county among the hospital doctors, who had publicly blamed the mode of treatment observed towards the patients, and spoken of another which he had seen practised with eminent success.
>
> 'Some impudent quack' said the general, 'who would force himself into business by bold assertions. Doctor Tourniquet and Doctor Lancelot are men of high reputation.'
>
> 'It is well known, that the ancient mode of treating the smallpox was to refuse the patient everything which nature urged him to desire; and in particular, to confine him to heated rooms, beds loaded with blankets, and spiced wine, when nature called for cold water and fresh air. A different mode of treatment had of late been adventured upon by some practitioners, who preferred reason the authority, and Gideon Gray had followed it with extraordinary success.'
>
> 'To treat a fever in this manner which tends to produce one, seems indeed to be adding fuel to fire.'
>
> 'It is—it is', said the lady 'Let us trust this young man . . . we shall give our darlings the comforts of fresh air and cold water, for which they are pining.' But the General remained undecided. 'Your reasoning' he said to Hartley, 'seems plausible; but still it is only hypothesis. What can you show to support your theory, in opposition to the general practice?'
>
> 'My own observation, 'replied the young man. 'Here is a memorandum-book of medical cases which I have witnessed. It contains twenty cases of smallpox, of which eighteen were recoveries.'. 'And the two others?' said the General. 'Terminated fatally' replied Hartley; 'We can as yet but partially disarm this scourge of the human race.'

This quotation reflects the difficulty in manging smallpox, before vaccination as a preventative measure became available, and the wide range of different methods used. The interaction between the doctors and the patients is also relevant. Who do I believe, and who will give the best treatment? The final remark, on the measurement of outcomes, is of particular interest as it begins to show the power of the collection of data in substantiating clinical practice, the beginning of evidenced-based medicine. It also answers the questions of the patients, as to who do I believe, and who will treat me most effectively.

A Window in Thrums (1889), J.M.Barrie[3]

> On the bump of the green round which the brae twists, at the top of the brae, and within cry of T'nowhead Farm, still stands a one-storey house, whose whitewashed walls, streaked with the discolouration that rain leaves, look yellow when the snow comes.

This is the opening paragraph of *A Window in Thrums* which describes the place where the family live and die and how through the window the life of the village can be observed. The house brings back memories of how the garret was papered with newspapers and how the yarn was used to stuff holes in the window. He reflects on the brae,

> Ah, that brae! The history of tragic little Thrums is sunk into it like the stones it swallows in the winter. We have all found the brae long and steep in the spring of life. Do you remember how the child you once were sat at the foot of it and wondered if a new world began at the top?

It represents a range of stories and events from small town Scotland at the end of the 19th century, well exemplified in one story called 'Waiting for the doctor'.[4]

The story begins with Jess, the mother, in bed as she cries to her daughter 'Leeby' who goes to discover that her mother is not well. 'It's diphtheria!' she says. The narrator does not reply because 'ever since this malady left me a lonely dominie, diphtheria has been a knockdown word for me. Jess had discovered a great white spot on her throat. I knew the symptoms.' They argue about what to do, whether she should eat something, but they decide that they should send for the doctor. She won't have the doctor at first, but Leeby eventually goes to fetch him and returns to say that he will be there in an hour, as he is away in the hills. They waited until night and watched the village go by. Hendry the husband at midnight climbs to the attic where the narrator has been sitting watching. 'She's waur.' They have been married for thirty-nine years, and he begins to recollect their life together. The night ends as they watch. 'Then came the terrible moment that precedes the day – the moment known to shuddering watchers by sick beds, when a chill wind cuts through the house, and the world without seems cold in death'.

The doctor arrives, his voice is heard, there is a painful silence, then Leeby laughs out loud. 'It's gone,' cries Jess; 'The white spot's gone! Ye juist touched it an' it's gone! Tell Hendry.' But Hendry did not need to be told. As Jess spoke I heard him say huskily: 'Thank God!'

The story is set in the days before vaccination and antibiotics, where the country doctor, delayed on his rounds, makes a diagnosis and effects a simple cure. The family's relief is clear.

A second short story, 'Dead these twenty years' reflects on grief.[5] Twenty years has passed since Joey ran down the brae to play. Jess his mother shook her staff fondly at him. A cart rumbled by, the driver nodding at the shaft. It rounded the corner and stopped suddenly, and then a woman screamed. A handful of men carried Joey's dead body to his mother, and that was the tragedy of Jess's life.

She still sits at the window watching for her son. On Sundays she cannot go to church, as it was then she was with Joey most. 'There was often a blessed serenity on her face when we returned.' She has another child, Jamie, but he does not quite fill the void, and she remembers Joey every day.

This is a poingant story of a mother's grief, and its long lasting effect on her and the family.

Peter Pan (1902), J.M.Barrie[6]

This remarkable story contains numerous references to health and medicine. For example, Mr Darling, the father, discusses expenses and says to the children:

'I have one pound seventeen here, and two and six in the office making two nine and six, with your eighteen and three makes three nine and seven, with five naught naught in my cheque book . . . Remember mumps, he warned her almost threateningly, and went off again. Mumps one pound, that is what I have put down but I daresay it will be more like thirty shillings. Don't speak – measles one five, German measles half a guinea makes two fifteen six-don't waggle your finger – whooping cough, say fifteen shillings' and so it went on.

Nana is the dog who acts as nursemaid:

She had a genius for knowing when a cough is a thing to have patience with and when it needs stocking round your throat. She believed to her last day in old-fashioned remedies like rhubarb leaf and made sounds of contempt over this new-fangled talk about germs, and so on.

Later in the story the Lost Boys are playing when they make a request to Wendy:

Then they all went on their knees and holding out their arms cried 'Oh Wendy lady, be our mother.' 'Ought I?' Wendy said all shining, 'Of course it's frightfully fascinating, but you see I am only a little girl. I have no real experience.'

Then to the key part of the story: Hook is the villain who tries to poison Peter Pan. We are told:

Lest he should be taken alive, Hook always carried about his person a dreadful drug, blended by himself of all the death-dealing rings that had come into his possession. These he had boiled down into a yellow liquid quite unknown to science, which was probably the most virulent poison in existence. Five drops he now added to Peter's cup

However Tinkerbell drinks it to save Peter Pan and she begins to die. Peter asks those who believe to clap their hands to stop Tinkerbell dying – and, thanks to the audience, she is saved.

From this play we can draw several incidents stand out. First, the reference here to the cost of infectious disease, and to one of the few notes on 'germs,' makes this a contemporary read. In addition Wendy is a girl and is expected to act like 'mother'. Finally, the mixing of powerful potions and the saving of Tinkerbell by the power of people willing her to get better, the power of human interaction, is the climax of the play.

Weir of Hermiston (1896), Robert Louis Stevenson[7]

This was Stevenson's last unfinished romance. In it he once again makes comments about the doctor, and the patient/doctor and patient/relative relationship, and telling the truth, in this instance surrounding infection.

Stevenson also mentions an old method of dealing with a sore throat, when he sees a prisoner with a 'piece of dingy flannel' pinned around his throat as part of the cure. In the days before antibiotics, this was common – I can recall it myself.

The doctor in question is the celebrated Professor James Gregory from Edinburgh. Archie is standing looking in the window of a book shop when a hand is laid on his arm and a voice says:

'My dear Mr Archie, you had better come and see me.' 'And why should I come to see you?' he replies.

'What makes you think that Hermis – my father would have missed me?'

'The doctor turned about and looked him all over with a clinical eye. A far more stupid man than Dr Gregory might have guessed the truth; but ninety-nine out of a hundred, even if they had been equally inclined to kindness, would have blundered by some touch of charitable exaggeration. The doctor was better inspired. He knew the father well; in that white face of intelligence and suffering, he divined something of the son; and he told without apology or adornment, the plain truth.'

'When you had the measles, Mr Archibald, you had them gey and ill; and I thought you were going to slip between my fingers,' he said. 'Well your father was anxious. How did I know it? Says you. Simply because I am a trained observer. The sign that I saw him make, ten thousand would have missed; and perhaps – perhaps, I say, because he is a hard man to judge . . .

it was this. One day I said to him 'Hermiston' said I, 'there's a change.' He never said a word, just glowered at me . . . like a wild beast. 'A change for the better,' said I. And I distinctly heard him take his breath' The doctor left no opportunity for anti-climax; nodding his cocked hat and repeating 'Distinctly'.

Here Stevenson describes the importance of clinical observation, expected of Dr Gregory, but also the way in which he communicates with the patient, with honesty and truth.

Healing wells and remedies

Over the centuries a range of wells and waters have been described as having healing properties. In Ruth and Frank Morris' book *Scottish Healing Wells* they describe around 150 wells.[8] Some of these are of considerable significance, such Scotlandwell in Perth and Kinross where Robert the Bruce is said to have been treated for leprosy. Some, the 'cloutie' wells, such as St Mary's well on the Black Isle, are covered in clouts, small cloths, tied to the surrounding trees to assist the healing. Several tales consider such wells or healing waters.

The Talisman, Sir Walter Scott[9]

It may seem strange to comment on a novel based on the medicine practices in the middle ages in this section on 19th century literature. Yet the novel raises a number of issues relevant to contemporary medicine and the importance placed in complementary medicine in the present day. This magic healing stone was eventually returned to Scotland. It is said that it is the Lee Penny and it remains in the possession of the Lockarts of Lee in Biggar in Lanarkshire.

One of the major themes of *The Talisman* is the healing of King Richard of England by an Arabian physician, El Hakim. The physician who has been befriended by Sir Kenneth, a Scottish knight, and his faithful hound Roswal who is also treated by the physician, turns out to be Suliman the Great. As part of the story El Hakim is asked about his art in front of the patient, to which he replies ' If thou knewest aught of medicine, thou wouldst be aware that physicians hold no counsel or debate in the sick chamber of their patient.' However, he does manage to heal King Richard using a magic stone and some potent drugs. The stone, inside a silver network, is placed in water for a few minutes and a change seems to occur. The patient is then asked to drink. Such magic and healing stones were well known and in St Fillans in Perth these stones are nicely displayed. The comment by El Hakim on not discussing the patient's condition in front of the patient is still relevant.

St. Ronan's Well, Sir Walter Scott[10]

The well, which is situated in Innerleithen in the Scottish Borders, is under the administration of a committee of members, chosen for their individual gifts. The narrator sets out the key players.

> First on the list stood the Man of Medicine, Dr Quentin Quackleben, who claimed the right to regulate medical matters at the spring, upon the principle which, of old, assigned the property of a newly discovered country to the buccaneer who committed the earliest piracy on its shores. The acknowledgement of the Doctor's merit, as having been the first to proclaim and vindicate the merits of these healing fountains, had occasioned his being universally installed First Physician and Man of Science, which last qualification he could apply to all purposes, from boiling an egg to the giving of a lecture. He was indeed qualified, like many of his profession, to spread both the bane and antidote before a dyspeptic patient, being as knowing a gastronome as Dr Redgill himself, or any other physician who has written for the benefit of the cuisine.

Dr Quackleben states proudly to one of his patients 'Fie, fie ma'am – I am no apothecary – I have my diploma from Leyden – a regular physician, madam.'

In the novel there are numerous references to Dr Quackleben trying hard to find additional fees from wealthy patients. He notes the size of their wallets, and makes sure he spends time with them. This link to patients and their spending power is a long lasting theme in medical practice.

The reference to Leyden is of particular importance as it was the leading medical school in Europe in the early 18th century, and its alumni from Scotland founded the Edinburgh Medical School, which led the way to its prominence in the second half of that century.

Johnny Gibb of Gushetneuk in the Parish of Pyketillum (1880), William Alexander[11]

In the district where Johnny Gibb lived they believed in the Walls (wells), old and young. Elderly people, male and female, went to Macduff to benefit by the bracing effects of sea-bathing, combined with a course more or less rigorous of seawater taken internally, followed up by the mineral water of Tarlair; sturdy bairns were taken thither in troops for the cure of 'scabbit faces and sic like'; youths and maidens, whose complaints seemed often not of a deadly nature, went to the wells as they could contrive to get; Jamie Hogg went there for the benefit of his 'sair een'; Peter Tough to mitigate the rheumatics.

The time is June 1839 and Johnny Gibb is preparing to set out on his annual journey to the 'Walls' (Wells) at Macduff. He is preparing the cart with his servant and the time is 4.30am.

Johnny Gibb was the tacksman of Gushetneuk . . . and he and his wife had spent the greater part of a very industrious lifetime on the place. Mrs Gibb, in personal appearance looked to be a woman somewhere approaching sixty, in an exceedingly good state of preservation. Dumpy in figure, inclining slightly to obesity in condition, and with cheeks of the exact hue of a high coloured apple . . . she was indeed nervish and apt to take drows (an attack of illness or anxiety). Hence this yearly resort to the Wells of Macduff, renowned for their restorative and invigorating virtues, had come to be a necessity for her. When Johnny Gibb had got the neeps doon, he took his carts to the mill-dam, had them backed into the water, where they were well soaked and scrubbed clean . . . and then one of the first things ordinarily, was to prepare for the usual journey to the Wells.

The farm servants even were fain to follow the prevailing custom; and this, their belief, had not been discouraged by the physician in ordinary, the elder Dr Drogemweal. The doctor had a semi-military reputation . . . it was related of him how he would make the delinquent soldier drink a quart bottle of sea water by way of punishment, believing that, while the thing had a penal effect, it also conserved the man's constitution.

Such was the reputation of the Wells at Macduff in my day, but that is long ago; and to me the modern Macduff is a place all bit totally unknown.

The daily round was uniform and systematic. You were expected to drink the salt water as an aperient once in two days at least, and to bathe every day.

The water was drunk in the morning, the patients helping themselves out of the Moray Firth . . . and then walking along the beach to the valley of Tarlair where they supplemented the salt water by drinking of the mineral steam that discharged itself at the little well-house, covered with several large Caithness flags that stood there. There was a little house too, at the foot of the north bank, where a drop of whisky could be got somehow in cases of emergency, and when the patient got hoven with the liberal libations of the salt water previously swallowed, or where the taste lay strongly in that direction; but this was no part of the recognised regime.

Then about midday was the season for bathing. The women-perhaps I should say the ladies-bathed at the part nearest the town, and the men further eastward.

This is a wonderful description of the process and the belief in such wells in which the whole community takes part.

Kidnapped (1886), Robert Louis Stevenson[12]

This incident recognises the importance of herbal and folk remedies in the treatment of disease. At the beginning of the story David Balfour, the hero, is given a package as a present. It contains a number of things including a little piece of coarse yellow paper on which is written:

To make Lilly of the Valley Water
Take the flowers of lilly of the valley and distil them in a sack, and drink a spoonful or two as there is an occasion. It restores speech to those that

have the dumb palsy. It is good against the gout; it comforts the heart and strengthens the memory; and the flowers put in a glass, close stopped, and set into ane hill of ants for a month, then take it out, and you will find a liquor which comes from the flowers, which keep in a vial; it is good, ill or well, and whether man or woman.

And in the minister's own hand, was added: 'Likewise for sprain, rub it in; and for the cholic, a great spoonful in the hour.' The use of herbal remedies was common and for most the only treatment available.' The food taken is also described and the availability of exotics, even in the Highlands is clear.

'This servant had a good sized portmanteau strapped on his horse, and a net of lemons (to brew punch with) hanging at the saddle bow; as was often enough the custom with luxurious travellers in that part of the country.' (Appin)

Reflections on illness and dying

In the literature of 19th century Scotland there are a number of poems about being unwell and the prospect of dying. The few here represent a selection of what was a common topic about which to write.

'The Sick Child', Robert Louis Stevenson

This poem conveys the anxiety and concerns of a child, something that Stevenson must have experienced often. It also gives the comforting reply of the mother trying to reassure and encourage healing sleep:

> CHILD
> O Mother, lay your hand on my brow!
> O mother, mother, where am I now?
> Why is this room so gaunt and great?
> Why am I lying awake so late?

217

MOTHER
Fear not at all: the night is still.
Nothing is here that means you ill –
Nothing but lamps the whole town through,
And never a child awake but you.

CHILD
Mother, mother, speak low in my ear
Some of the things are so great and near,
Some are so small and far away
I have a fear that I cannot say,
What have I done, and what do I fear
And why are you crying, mother dear?

MOTHER
Out in the city, sounds begin
Thank the kind God, the carts come in!
And hour or two more, and God is so kind
The day shall be blue in the window-blind,
Then shall my child go sweetly asleep,
And dream of the birds and the hills of sheep.[13]

'Land o' the Leal', Lady Caroline Nairne (1766–1845)

Lady Caroline wrote a large number of songs including 'Caller Herring' and 'Will ye no' come back again'. She also wrote this beautiful sad poem, 'The Land of the Leal'[14] – the land of the blessed after death, the land of the faithful. This poem reflects her last words to her husband as she is dying:

Land o' the Leal
I'm wearin' awa, John
Like snaw-weaths in thaw, John
I'm wearin' awa
    To the land O' the leal

There's nae sorrow there, John
There's nae cauld nor care, John
The day is aye fair
    In the land o' the leal

Sae dear's the joy was bought, John
Sae free the battle fought, John
That sinfu' man e'er brought
    To the land o' the leal.

O, dry your glist'nin e'e, John!
My saul langs to be free, John
And angels beckon me
    To the land o' the leal.

O, haud ye leal and true, John!
Your day is wearin' thro', John
And I'll welcome you
    To the land o' the leal

Now fare-ye-weel, my ain John
This warld's care are vain, John
We'll meet, and we'll be fain John [affectionate]
    In the land o' the leal.'

This poem covers the issues around a peaceful death, and the battle fought and won. She will have no pain or sorrow in the Land o' the Leal and she thinks ahead, to when they will met again and, which according to her faith, she can welcome him there.

The House with the Green Shutters, George Douglas Brown (1869–1902)[15]

The House wtih the Green Shutters provides a quite different setting and disease and it is a remarkable description of the problems of breast cancer. Two women discuss the problem:

Janet's heart was rent for her brother, but the frenzy on her mother killed sorrow with a new fear.

'Janet!' smiled Mrs Gourlay, with insane soft interest, 'Janet! D'ye mind yon nicht langsyne when your faither came in wi' a terrible look in his een and struck me in the breist? Ay,' she whispered hoarsely, staring at the fire, 'he struck me in the breist. But I didna ken what it was for, Janet ... No,' she shook her head, 'he never told me what it was for.'

'Ay, mother,' whispered Janet, 'I have mind o't.'

'Weel, an abscess o' some kind formed – I kenna weel what it was, but it gathered and broke, and gathered and broke, till my breist's near eaten awa wi't. Look!' she cried, tearing open her bosom, and Janet's head flung back in horror and disgust.

'O mother!' she panted, 'was it that that the wee clouts were for?'

'Ay, it was that,' said her mother. 'Mony a clout I had to wash, and mony a nicht I sat lonely by mysell, plaistering my withered breist. But I never let onybody ken,' she added with pride; 'na-a-a, I never let onybody ken. When your faither nipped me wi' his tongue it nipped me we' its pain, and, woman, it consoled me. 'Ay, ay,' I used to think; 'gibe awa, gibe awa; but I hae a freend in my breist that'll end it some day.' I likit to keep it to mysell. When it bit me it seemed to whisper I had a freend that nane o' them kenned o' - a freend that would deliver me! The mair he hadgered me, the closer I hugged it; and when my he'rt was br'akin I enjoyed the pain o't.'

The patient uses breast cancer as a way of dealing with many other problems and she knows that her cancer will be the one thing which will release her from the other difficulties in her life. It is a very powerful ending of a book which was written in 1901. It is relevant to note that Sir George Beatson at the Western Infirmary Glasgow (1848–1908) wrote on this subject in 1896 when he published a paper entitled 'On the treatment of incurable cancer of the mamma: Suggestions of a new method of treatment'.[16] This proposed the removal of the ovaries in such patients with significant remission of the disease.

Disorders of the mind

The 19th century saw a greater recognition of mental disorders and at the same time the building of mental asylums for those with mental disease. Charcot (1825–1893) in France had pioneered hypnosis and the study of hysteria. By the end of the century Freud had begun psychoanalysis and in 1899 published *The interpretation of Dreams*. The three extracts set out here cover some of the issues involved.

The Private Memoirs and Confessions of a Justified Sinner (1824), James Hogg (1770–1835)[17]

Sometimes known as the Ettrick Shepherd, Hogg, after reading Tam o'Shanter, determined to become a poet. Access to a library was available and he published numerous poems.

James Hogg's tale *The Private Memoirs and Confessions of a Justified Sinner* is a disturbing but powerful book of how an individual driven by religious certainty as being one of the elect carries out a series of crimes and acts of depravity, though it received little critical acclaim at the time. The book is written in the first person and main character is accompanied in this by a person whose personality and appearance change. Eventually it becomes so bad that the individual commits suicide. As a description of serious illness, perhaps related to alcohol and personality disorder it is very powerful indeed. The comments by Professor Robin Murray, until recently Professor of Psychiatry at the Maudesley in London are relevant (personal communication). His views on this are as follows, though it is worth pointing out that not everything is as it seems in this book:

> I don't think one can conclude that the main character exhibits the classic signs of one particular psychiatric disorder. Rather, at different points in the manuscript there are astute descriptions of aspects of different conditions. It is clear that, as a child, the 'sinner' already had difficulty in relating to both

children and his teachers, and as an adolescent, paranoid traits led him to be particularly entranced by a doctrine with explicit rules concerning right-eous living and deliverance, and which condemned those who transgressed he rules to exclusion from 'the elect'.

Some might conclude that the description of the 'sinner's' companion indi-cates that the 'sinner' was hallucinated, and thus schizophrenic. However, schizophrenic hallucinations are almost invariably auditory and it is very rare to come across a patient who will so clearly describe the repeated appear-ance of a hallucinatory figure. Furthermore, the text indicates that, at vari-ous points, others have also seen the 'sinner's' companion, and it is unlikely that visual hallucinations would be shared. Certainly, however, the 'sinner' is psychotic at times, and obviously much of his reasoning is paranoid.

One can see how the solitary life that the 'sinner' leads results in his having insufficient social interactions with anyone to test the reality of his internal dialogues with the prince, i.e. he has no external correction of his increasingly extravagant delusional ideas. Later in the text, after the 'sinner' becomes the 'elect' and gets access to the wine cellar, he relates a long period when he cannot recollect the events of some two months during which he indulged in various debauched acts. This might be a form of dissociation from the 'evil' deeds that he has committed (greed, sex etc.) but a more likely explanation would be a continued alcoholic binge, with blackouts and loss of memory. Later, one can conceive of some of the events nearer the end of the book (e.g. the struggle with the spider's web) as the 'sinner' experiencing delirium tremens during alcohol withdrawal. The final period is obviously one of increasing depression, guilt and despair. Phrases such as my 'vitals have all been torn' and my 'soul racked and tormented' are quite common amongst patients with psychotic depression.[18]

Throughout the book there are fascinating illustrations of how solitary and paranoid individuals become increasingly divorced from reality and carry out, and indeed justify to themselves, acts which the rest of us regard as heinous. One can see echoes in the book of some of the modern lone mass murderers. This is a unique book, dark and troubling, and with a special insight into mental health problems.

Jekyll and Hyde, Robert Louis Stevenson (1850–1894)[19]

Mental disease is difficult to deal with and this story shows the devastating impact of split personalities. *Jekyll and Hyde* is a classic. Here Stevenson describes how an individual can change from one person into another, he uses a chemical means to do it, but the novel makes clear that Hyde and Jekyll were the different sides of the same person. Hyde sets out the problem:

> That night I had come to the fatal cross roads. Had I approached my discovery in a more noble spirit, had I risked the experiment while under the empire of generous or pious aspirations, all must have been otherwise, and from these agonies of death and birth I had come forth an angel instead of a fiend. The drug had no discriminating action; it was neither diabolical nor divine; it but shook the doors of the prison-house of my disposition; and, like the captives of Phillippi, that which stood within ran forth. At that time my virtue slumbered; my evil, kept awake by ambition, was alert and swift to seize the occasion; and the thing that was projected was Edward Hyde. Hence, although I had now two characters as well as two appearances, one was wholly evil, and the other was still the old Henry Jekyll, that incongruous compound of whose reformation and improvement I had already learned to despair. The movement was thus wholly toward the worse.

He continues,

> Between these two, I now felt I had to choose. My two natures had memory in common, but all other faculties were most unequally shared between them. Jekyll (who was composite) now with the most sensitive, apprehensions, now with a greedy gusto, projected and shared in the pleasures and adventures of Hyde; but Hyde was indifferent to Jekyll, or but remembered him as the mountain bandit remembers the cavern in which he conceals himself from pursuit. Jekyll had more than a father's interest; Hyde had

more than a son's indifference. To cast in my lot with Jekyll was to die to those appetites which I had long secretly indulged and had of late begun to pamper. To cast it in with Hyde was to die to a thousand interests and aspirations, and to become, at a blow and for ever, despised and friendless. The bargain might appear unequal; but there was still another, consideration in the scales; for while Jekyll would suffer smartingly in the fires of abstinence, Hyde would be not even conscious of all that he had lost. Strange as my circumstances were, the terms of this debate are as old and common-place as man; much the same inducements and alarms cast the die for any tempted and trembling sinner; and it fell out with me, as it falls with so vast a majority of my fellows, that I chose the better part, and was found wanting in the strength to keep to it.

This is a powerful book exposing again the difficulties of diagnosing and treating such an extreme clinical problem, compounded by the evil nature of Jekyll who had the ability and will do carry out such deeds. There are times when medicine has reached its limits and there are no quick solutions or easy answers, hence the importance of documentation and research.

'The City of the Dreadful Night', James Thomson (BV) (1834–1882)[20]

This is a remarkable poem about depression and melancholia, written in 1880. Thomson sets out at the start to why he writes this poem:

> Because it gives some sense of power and passion
> In helpless innocence to try to fashion
>   Our woe in living words howe'er uncouth.

In setting the scene he writes:

> Surely I write not for the hopeful young
> Or those who deem their happiness of worth
> Or such as pasture and grow fat among
> The shows of life and feel nor doubt nor dearth,

> Or pious spirits with a god above them
> To sanctify and glorify and love them
> Or sages who foresee a heaven on earth.

But he writes for:

> If anyone cares for the weak words here written
> It must be someone desolate, Fate – smitten
> Whose faith and hopes are dead, and who would die.

Someone who:

> Will understand the speech and feel a stir
> Of fellowship in all-disastrous fight
> I suffer mute and lonely, yet another
> Uplifts his voice to let me know a brother
> Travels the same wild paths though out of sight.

Thus though the poem is depressing, his writing of it has given him 'power and passion' and he hopes that it will connect with others with similar problems.

He then describes what depression feels like using a series of illustrations of the city. 'The City is of night; perchance of death', reflecting his moods, his inability to sleep: 'The City is of night, but not of sleep', his conscious thoughts and lack of hope. As he walks round the city, memories are invoked, but each time he returns to 'dead Faith, dead Love, dead Hope' and fear is everywhere. He is alone with his melancholia:

> I never knew another man on earth
> But had some joy and solace in his life
> Some chance of triumph in the dreadful strife:
> My doom has been unmitigated dearth.

And he does not ask for much:

> And yet I asked no splendid dower, no spoil
> Of sway or fame or rank or even wealth
> But homely love with common food and health
> And nightly sleep to balance daily toil.

He briefly mentions 'opium visions' but he then wakes to 'Real night'. He thinks he might have one chance to be happy, but this is 'frustrated from my birth.' And his 'wine of life is poison mixed with gall.' This is an interesting reference as in the Hippocratic 'Humours' depression/melancholia is represented by black bile which originates in the gall bladder. Indeed black bile from the ancient Greek is '*melas*' (dark) *and* '*khole*' (bile) melancholy.

His thoughts on suicide are also relevant:

> The mighty river flowing dark and deep
> With ebb and flood from the remote sea-tides
> Vague-sounding through the City's sleepless sleep
> Is named the river of suicides;
> For night by night some lorn wretch overweary
> And shuddering from the future yet more dreary,
> Within its cold secure oblivion hides.

> One plunges from a bridge's parapet
> As if by some blind and sudden frenzy hurled:
> Another wades in slow with purpose set
> Until the waters above him are furled;
> Another in a boat with dream like motion
> Glides drifting down into the desert ocean
> To starve or sink from out the desert world.

He then imagines the Winged Woman in Albrecht Durer's engraving. She leans forward, a clasped book on her lap, and the instruments of science around her, and a bat flying away with 'Melancholia' written on its wings.

There have been numerous interpretations of Durer's engraving. Some see it as the woman reflecting, waiting for inspiration, and it is interesting that the bat, with 'Melancholia' is flying away. Melancholia was sometimes attributed to students or seekers after knowledge and the period before inspiration. Others see it as a picture of depression, and the inability to do anything in spite of all the instruments of science being available to her.

The final few lines are ambiguous and return to the very beginning of the poem, and pick up on the engraving:

> Her subjects often gaze up to her there:
> The strong to drink new strength of iron endurance
> The weak new terrors; all, renewed assurance
> And confirmation of the old despair.

Is there any space here for hope? In helping others does he himself improve? Thomson's own life story is relevant here. James Thomson (1834–1882) was born in Port Glasgow, but after the death of his father he was sent to London where he was raised in an orphanage, and as a result he spoke with a London accent. He made friends with Charles Bradlaugh who began a weekly paper, The *National Reformer* and Thomson submitted stories, essays and poems to it. He wrote under the pseudonym *Bysshe Vanolis* (BV) to distinguish himself from an earlier writer with the same name. His own final years were difficult with problems of insomnia, alcoholism and depression. He died at the age of 47.

There are numerous references throughout the history of medicine to melancholia, including in the *Canon of Medicine* by Avicenna, and in particular by Robert Burton in his large work *The Anatomy of Melancholy* published in 1621. Relevant, are Burton's comments on the role of the arts, and in particular music and dance in improving the mental state. Depression remains a significant clinical problem to the present day.

Conclusions

This chapter has dealt with some of the illnesses which are recorded in the literature and the relevant treatment. Infection is a key problem, though it is interesting that neither cholera nor typhus are discussed, although there were well recorded epidemics throughout the century. This is a topic which will be raised again in the next chapter.

The treatments are limited, and there is little on surgical management, yet this was rapidly transforming the outcome of care during this time. Anaesthesia is mentioned in 'Rab and His Friends' discussed in the previous chapter, because it was not used, and antisepsis is considered, again in the previous chapter, in relation to antiseptic dressings. (*A Doctor of the Old School*). It should be recalled that Queen Victoria used chloroform to help deliver her 7th child in 1853. There are no links to the major developments in bacteriology and pathology. Folk remedies predominate, and there is little evidence of their effectiveness, or indeed of the healing wells and waters. The change to the 20th century is thus all the more striking, where realism, advances in treatment, descriptions of disease, are all openly discussed, as we shall see. The next chapter on social conditions and lifestyle, will also identify the lack of realism in the writings, especially in the Victorian period (1858–1901). Some of the possible reasons for this will be discussed later.

On the other hand those writings on sickness and dying have a more long lasting and contemporary feel. They describe the feelings and concerns of individuals, and the story on cancer (*The House of the Green Shutters*) is a particularly poignant one, noting the wishes of the patient that death will remove all her troubles. This terrain reflects some of the poems previously noted in the 18th century. Such feelings are the same today and the debates on assisted suicide continue to raise difficult ethical questions.

Notes

1   John Galt, *Annals of the Parish*. The World's Classics (Oxford: OUP, 1986).

2   A.K. Chalmers, *The Health of Glasgow 1818–1925: An Outline* (Glasgow: Corporation of Glasgow, 1930); A.K. Chalmers, *Public Health Administration in Glasgow: a Memorial Volume of the Writings of James Burn Russell* (Glasgow: James Maclehose and Sons, 1905); C.F. Brockington, *Public Health in the 19th Century* (Edinburgh: E and S Livingstone, 1965); Michael Flynn, ed., *Scottish Population History from the 17th Century to the 1930s* (Cambridge: Cambridge University Press, 1977).

3   J.M. Barrie, *A Window In Thrums* (London: Hodder and Stoughton, 1937).

4   Ibid, 'Waiting for the Doctor', pp. 39–50.

5   Ibid, 'Dead These Twenty Years', , pp. 63–76.

6   J.M. Barrie, *Peter Pan* (London: Vintage Classics, 2009).

7   Robert Louis Stevenson, *Weir of Hermiston* (London: Penguin Books, 1979).

8   Ruth and Frank Morris, *Scottish Healing Wells* (Sandy: The Alethea Press, 1982).

9   Walter Scott, *The Talisman* (London: J.M. Dent, 1980).

10 Walter Scott, *St. Ronan's Well* (London: The Caxton Publishing Co., 1903).

11 William Alexander, *Johnny Gibb of Gushetneuk in the Parish of Pyketillum* (Edinburgh: David Douglas, 1881).

12 Robert Louis Stevenson, *Kidnapped* (Edinburgh: Polygon, 2007).

13 'The Sick Child', Stevenson, *Underwoods and Ballads*, pp. 39–40.

14 Lady Caroline Nairne, 'The Land of the Leal', *The Penguin Book of Scottish Verse*, ed. by Tom Scott (London: Penguin Books, 1970), pp. 361–62.

15 George Douglas Brown, *The House with the Green Shutters* (Edinburgh: The Mercat Press, 1986).

16 Sir George Beatson, 'On the Treatment of Incurable Cancer of the Mamma: Suggestions of a New Method of Treatment', *The Lancet*, 2 (1896), 104–7.

17 James Hogg, *The Private Memoirs and Confessions of a Justified Sinner* (London: Penguin Books, 1983).

18 Personal communication with Professor Robin Murray.

19 Robert Louis Stevenson, *The Strange Case of Dr Jekyll and Mr Hyde* (London: William Heinemann, 1924).

20 James Thomson (B.V.), *The City of Dreadful Night* (Glasgow: Kennedy and Boyd, 2008).

CHAPTER 15

Social conditions and lifestyle

Oh, thou demon Drink, thou fell destroyer;
Thou curse of society, and its greatest annoyer.
What hast thou done to society, let me think?
I answer thou hast caused the most of ills, thou demon Drink.

William McGonagall

I have already demonstrated that social conditions, which include housing, employment, lifestyle, and family circumstances, are shown in literature to be relevant in determining health. During the 19th century there were enormous changes to such conditions, especially in the larger towns in the west of Scotland, as the population grew and industrialisation became established. The housing situation was difficult and slums rapidly developed. There was inward migration from other parts of Scotland and from Ireland, and such changes had a major impact on health. Overcrowding was rife and the practice of 'ticketing' was introduced in some places whereby a 'ticket' was placed outside a dwelling indicating the maximum number of people allowed to live in the rooms. The rooms were regularly inspected and people moved out if too many were found. As an example, the population of Glasgow rose from 77,385 in 1801 to 147,043 in 1821.[1] The conditions were well recorded in the photographs of Thomas Annan in Glasgow and David Octavius Hill and Robert Adamson in Edinburgh later in the century.

While there is significant evidence of change to social conditions throughout the century, the literature of the period does not always reflect this. There are no major writers who use the topics of poverty, alcohol or housing conditions, quite different from the great novels of industrialisation in the 20th century, indeed different from writers such as Dickens and Disraeli in England in the 19th century. The Kailyard and the rural environment tend to dominate. In other areas there were outspoken voices, notably in the church, and in particular Thomas Chalmers, whose writings on poverty provided an important catalyst for change.[2] This lack of realism may also be reflected in the paintings of the time and the lack of detective novels in the Scottish literature, though not in the emerging art of photography. These are some of the issues which will be discussed later.

There are a few poems which refer to alcohol and its dangers, but little on drugs, though opium taking was common. There is almost nothing on tobacco and cigarette smoking, and this will be illustrated later.

For convenience, this chapter is divided into a series of sections, though it should be clear that they are all interconnected: the changing city, food and nutrition, alcohol, tobacco, poverty and industrialisation and water quality.

The changing city

At the beginning of the 19th century Glasgow, the city at the heart of this change, could be described in an idyllic way.

'Glasgow' (1803), John Mayne (1759–1836)[3]

Mayne was born and educated in Dumfries and was a journalist there before moving to Glasgow. He published a number of poems, including 'Logan Braes', similar to that of Burns' 'Logan waters'.

'Glasgow'

Look through the town! The houses here
Like noble palaces appear;
A' things the face of gladness wear
The market's thrang
Business is brisk, and a's asteer
The streets alang

'Tween ane and twa, wi' gawsy air,
The Merchants to the Cross repair
And tho' they shine like Nabobs there

> Yet weil I wat,
> Commerce engages a' their care.
> And a' their chat.
>
> Thir wylie birkies trade to a'
> The Indies and America;
> Whate'er can mak' ae penny taw,
> Or raise their pride
> Is wafted to the Broomielaw
> On bonny Clyde.

Glasgow, the 'dear green place', a city of fields and orchards, a rural place on the banks of the Clyde, an easily forded river; it is also a merchant city with wealth and links to the Americas and the City of the Tobacco Lords. This is another link to cigarette and tobacco consumption (much like Liverpool), which needs some thought. It is a clean place, with open spaces and good conversation.

Contrast this with a poem written forty years later. This extract from the poem begins to describe the squalor and the dirt which changed the city for ever.

'How we spent the Sabbath Day' (Anonymous 1846):

> Our's is a wee dark unco crowded house
> Cramm'd in a strait an' foul overcrowded street;
> We can afford nae better, an' wham loose
> Frae six days toil, I homeward turn my feet
> I'm glad at heart an' grateful; as is meet
> For then God's hallow'd day comes roun' again
> Blest the day of rest! [4]

A quite different scene is painted; dirt, narrow streets and overcrowding, and also the importance of the Sabbath for rest.

Meanwhile John Galt is writing about a quite different rural situation, and exposes some of the social differences which occur.

The Provost (1822), John Galt

Written in 1822 this describes the events in the political life of small town Scotland.[5] It provides, like the *Annals of the Parish,* glimpses of life, social behaviour and health.

For example, the terrible story of Jeanie Gaisling is worth noting. She becomes pregnant and probably murders her bastard bairn. After the mid-wife has left she is discovered with the bairn black in the face in the bed beside her. She is tried, found guilty and sentenced not only to be hanged, but ordered to be executed in the town, and her body to be given to the doctors to make an atomy (anatomical dissection).

The problems of poverty are clearly set out. Food was scarce and getting expensive, and the plight of women in particular is well described by the Provost.

Many a decent auld woman that had patiently eked out the slender thread of a weary life with her wheel, in privacy, her scant and want known only to her maker, was seen going from door to door, with the salt tear in her e'e, and looking in the face of the pitiful, being as yet unacquainted with the language of beggary; but the worst sight of all, was the two bonny bairns, drest in their best, of a genteel demeanour, going from house to house, like the hungry babes in the wood . . . they told me their mother was lying sick and ill at home. They were the orphans of a broken merchant from Glasgow, and, with their mother, had come to our town the week before, without knowing where else to seek their meat.

In 1813 the main character in the novel is chosen as Provost for the third time, and

at the special request of My Lord the Earl, who being in ill health, had been advised by the faculty of doctors in London to try the medicinal virtues of the air and climate of Sicily . . . with an understanding that he should hold the post of Honour for two years chiefly in order to bring to a conclusion different works that the town had then.

These short extracts give a sense of what was happening in the town, the social structure and some health-related issues. Poverty was a major issue and will be a recurring theme in this 19th century section.

During the 19th century there were a number of 'improvements' to city and town planning and one of the most famous was the development in New Lanark (1786) by Robert Owen (1771–1858) and David Dale (1739–1806), who by education, work and religion vowed to change society.

As an example of a novel related to this, *Margaret Maitland* by Margaret Oliphant (1828–1897), is one of the most interesting.[6] Margaret Oliphant was one of the most extraordinary woman writers of her day. Born in Scotland, she moved to Liverpool and then London and during her life time wrote around ninety books. They are remarkably easy to read, full of good sense, and reflect the values of Victorian culture. *The Chronicles of Carlingford* are perhaps most well known and are set in England. However, one of her earliest novels, *Margaret Mailtand,* reflects the changing world in early Victorian Scotland. It is set in a small town within a day's ride of Edinburgh, and is the story of a spinster who looks after a young woman and the complex interactions between her and the community. It is beautifully written and gives some fascinating insights into Scottish life at the time. For example, after a wedding, 'dreaming cake' is distributed, to be put under the pillows of those who are yet to be married.

From a health point of view, however, the most interesting part is the story of the local young laird. He is introduced to the village which has at one end of it an area which is poor and destitute and rather run down. The dialogue describes the issues which confront the village, and the potential remedies chosen to make improvements to the quality of life of its people.

Mr Allan's eyes shone out a light like the sparkle of a fire. 'Pestilence and violence, dirt and poverty!' he cried out. 'Splendid, Miss Maitland, and on my own estate too; almost too good news to be true! We'll have at it immediately! I shall ride down today, and begin. Cruive End! There is an expressive odour about the very name. But there, now, you are looking grave again. I have surely said nothing wrong just now.'

He, therefore, has a plan to completely change the village, rebuild the houses and in particular to encourage the men of the village to attend a series of morally edifying lectures on poetry and philosophy. As the story develops it becomes clear that this 'top-down' approach is not effective; he disturbs village life and it is no longer as it should be. The young laird, together with Margaret Maitland, recognises the folly of this so he makes amends by engaging a Glasgow merchant who sets up a mill just outside the village. He then plans a model village. This, as the story concludes, begins to be a success and provides employment and opportunity. It is very much the story of Robert Owen and David Dale in New Lanark. The fact that this should be well described in fictional literature, with the consequences of 'top-down' or 'bottom-up' being so clearly outlined represents the great insight of Margaret Oliphant. Her writing deserves greater attention. The dialogue, introduced by Mr Allen, sets out the new venture proposed:

'Oh! Mr Bogle will expound my last and grandest shceme to you tomorrow, aunt,' said Mr Allen, with a motion of his head towards his companion, who was a man of a douce and sensible aspect. 'I am about to commence business, in behoof of myself and my respectable tenantry of Cruive End, as – don't be horrified – a cotton spinner!'

'A cotton spinner!' cried out both Mary and my sister and me, in one breath. 'Verily,' said Mr Allen, laughing, 'nothing less. And this water of ours, which, like myself, has been idling all its life, must, like myself also, learn to be useful in its maturer years. I am perfectly serious, aunt. Mr Bogle is the apostle of a system of reform as different as possible from that of Novimundy; a system which does not undertake to make Cruive End idlers sentimental florists and makers of poetry, but, if they choose, independent men'.

The story continues:

It is a matter of thankfulness to me, to say here, that the mill in Cruive End has thriven in an uncommon manner, and the new generation give glints of a better disposition, and at least, in an outward and carnal way, are like to live a more creditable life than their forbears, besides that the Kirk among them is well attended, and I doubt not, the sowing of the good seed will be blessed

The vision of Owen and Dale set out in novel form, with an appropriate ending.

In the North East of Scotland J.M. Barrie was writing about Kirriemuir in *A Window in Thrums* and *Auld licht Idylls*, describing life in a small town.

Auld Licht Idylls is the story of the schoolmaster, the dominie, who has returned to Thrums.[7] There are a series of short stories two of which are relevant to this chapter. In the first, the narrator tells the story of the fight of Cabbylatch, which occurred some years before, dimly remembered as the Meal Mobs. There was a cry all over the country for bread, not the fine bread that we know, but something much coarser, and people had begun to forget the taste of meal. Potatoes were the chief sustenance and when the crop failed starvation gripped them. The people climbed up the sides of carts of meal and tearing the sacks open, devoured it in handfuls. They then took it into the market and sold it; a remarkable story of people, some of whom were starving, taking action to relief the problem for themselves.

The second is the establishment of a literary club. The ministers do not like it, perhaps because one of the questions frequently asked is 'Is literature necessarily immoral?' It's a fighting club, and on Friday night:

. . . a few respectable god-fearing people, dandered to the Town House to take part in the debates.' The attendance was greatest on dark nights and reading an essay on William Pitt lead to the club being bundled out of the Town House. There was little drinking at these meetings, for the members knew what they were talking about, and your mind had to gallop to keep up with the flow of reasoning. The literature was wide and varied, and members read papers to each other.

Such book clubs, or literary societies, still thrive and for medical students they provide another way of viewing health and medicine. Indeed this book began as a group of medical students listening reading and talking about books.

Food and nutrition

This is a topic which is well covered in the literature, and the link to the Americas accounts for some of the more exotic food found in Scotland in this period.

For Example, Sir Walter Scott in *Rob Roy* (1818) describes some of the health interest related to the food eaten in Scotland. Here is an exchange between two characters in the book.

'There's no such plenty of good cheer in your country, my good friend,' I replied, 'as to tempt you to sit so late at it.'

'Hout sir, ye ken little about Scotland; it's no for want of gude vivers-the best of fish, flesh and fowl hae we, by sybos, ingans, turneeps and other garden fruits. But we hae mense and discretion, and are moderate of our mouths . . . Even their fast days – they ca' it fasting when they hae the best o' sea fish frae Hartlepool and Sunderland, by land carriage, forbye trouts, grilses, and salmon'

And there is more advice.

'Is it not concluded, sir' replied the magistrate, 'man requires digestion as well as food, and I protest I cannot have benefit from my victuals, unless I am allowed two hours of quiet leisure, intermixed with harmless mirth, and a moderate circulation of the bottle.'

Annals of the Parish (1821), John Galt

The descriptions of the food eaten are fascinating. From Jamaica and the West Indies, sugar and coffee are brought home, and amongst the kail-stocks and the cabbages they had planted grozet (gooseberry) and berry bushes; which two things happening together encouraged the fashion for making jams and jellies began. Jelly was regarded as an excellent medicine for a sore throat, jam for a cough or a cold, or shortness of breath.

In 1788 he is invited to dine, and mutton and fowls which twenty years ago could not have been gotten for love or money were served together with bottles of red and white wine.

Alcohol – the demon drink

Alcohol was a major problem throughout this century, and indeed in the coming ones. It was a century of the Temperance Movement and legislation and with high political stakes. For example in Dundee as late as 1922, Winston Churchill was defeated in an election by Edwin Scrimgeour who stood in a Temperance/Prohibitionist Ticket.

William McGonagall, himself from Dundee writes beautifully on a variety of subjects, but from a health point of view his poem on 'The Demon Drink' takes a lot of beating:[8]

> Oh, thou demon Drink, thou fell destroyer;
> Thou curse of society, and its greatest annoyer.
> What hast thou done to society, let me think?
> I answer thou hast caused the most of ills, thou demon Drink.
>
> Thou causeth the mother to neglect her child,
> Also the father to act as he were wild,
> So that he neglects his loving wife and family dear,
> By spending his earnings foolishly on whisky, rum, and beer.
>
> And after spending his earnings foolishly he beats his wife -
> The man that promised to protect her during life -
> And so that man would if there was no drink in society,
> For seldom a man beats his wife in a state of sobriety.

'The Drunkard's Raggit Wean', James P. Crawford (1825-1887)

This is one of the most powerful poems related to alcohol. According to the introduction to this poem in *The Glasgow Poets* James P. Crawford composed this poem in 1855 while listening to the sermon in church. It was first published in *The Crystal Fount,* a temperance song book, with 33,000 copies sold in a year and over 17,000 sold as single sheets. A Miss Dougall sang the piece in Glasgow City Hall to great effect. Crawford was born in the Ayrshire village of Catrine, and moved to Glasgow to become a tailor. He had a keen sense of humour and loved a joke. He died in Ibrox in Govan in 1887 and this poem sums up the long-term and very modern issues of drunkenness.

'The Drunkard's Raggit Wean'

A wee bit raggit laddie gangs wan'rin through the street
Wadin' mang the snaw wi' his wee hackit feet,
Shiverin' i' the cauld blast, greetin' wi' the pain –
Wha's the poor wee laddie callan? He's a drunkard's raggit wean.

He stan's at ilka door, an' keeks wi' wistfu' e'e
To see the crowd aroun' the fire a' laughin' loud wi' glee;
But he daurna venture ben, though his heart be e'er sae fain
For he mauna play wi' ither bairns, the drunkard's raggit wean.

Oh, see the wee bit bairnie, his heart is unco fu',
The sleet is blawin' cauld, and he's droukit through and through;
He's speerin' for his mither, an' he won'ers where she's gane;
But oh! His mither she forgets her puir wee raggit wean.

He kens nae faither's love, and he kens nae mither's care,
To soothe his wee bit sorrows, or kame his tautit hair,
To kiss him when he waukens, or smooth his bed at e'en
An' oh! He fears his faither's face, the drunkard's raggit wean.

Oh, pity the wee laddie, sae guileless an'sae young!
The oath that lea's the faither's lips'll settle on his tongue
An' sinfu' words his mither speaks his infant lips 'll stain
For oh! There's nane to guide the bairn, the drunkard's raggit wean.

Then surely we micht try an' turn that sinfu' mither's heart
An' try to get his faither at act a faither's part
An' mak' them lea' the drunkard's cup, an' never taste again,
An' cherish wi' a parents' care their puir wee raggit wean.[9]

This presents a powerful and compelling case for acting on the problem of alcohol abuse; the effect on families and social order, the impact on children, the loss of earnings and of lack of money on all around the drunkard.

'Oor Location', Janet Hamilton (1795–1873)

Born in Carshill in Lanarkshire, she married at thirteen and raised a large family. Her poems reflect the conditions of the industrial world and mining communities in Lanarkshire and emphasises the alcohol problem, even in women. The poem considers where the family live, admidst factories and furnaces, and the 'dreadful curse of drinking':

'Oor Location'

A hunner funnels bleezin', reekin',
Coal an' ironstone charrin', smeekin [smoking)]
Navvies, miners, keepers, fillers,
Puddlers, rollers, iron millers;
Reestit, reekit raggit laddies,
Fireman, enginemen, an' paddies;
Boatmen, banksmen, rough an rattlin',
'Bout the wecht wi' colliers battling [weight]
Sweatin', searin', fechtin, drinkin';
Change-house bells and gill-stoup clinkin';
Police-ready men and willin'–
Aye at hand when stoups are fillin';
Clerks an' counter-loupers plenty [shop assistants]
Wi trim moustache and whiskers dainty
Chaps that winna staun at trifles!
Min' ye they can han'le rifles

   'Bout the wives in oor location
An' the lassies botheration
Some are decent, some are dandies
Some are gey wheen drucken randies [drunken foul mouthed]
Aye to neighbours houses sailin'
Greetin'bairns ahint then trailing

240

Gaun for nouther bread or butter
Juist to drink and rin the cutter! [get liquor from the pub]
O the dreadful curse o' drinkin'!
Men are ill, but, to my thinkin'
Leukin' through the drucken fock
There's a Jenny for ilk John
Oh the dool and desolation,
And the havock in the nation
Wrocht by dirty druken wives!
Oh hoo mony bairnies lives
Lost ilk year through their neglec'!
Like a millstone roun' the neck
O' the struggling, toilin' masses
Hing drucken wives an' wanton lasses
To see sae mony unwed mithers
Is sure a shame that taps a' ithers.[10]

This poem particularly emphasises the effect of alcohol on women and the implications for the children, and the issue of unmarried mothers.

Tobacco

Scotland has one of the highest cigarette smoking rates in the world, and the highest lung cancer mortality rates. Its link with the Americas, mainly through Glasgow, has already been noted. There is not much written about tobacco in the literature of Scotland. Tobacco was introduced to Britain shortly after the discovery of America, and initially smoking was by pipe or cigar. It took off during the Crimean war when the Russians began to roll tobacco in newspapers rather than on tobacco leaf. The dangers of cigarette smoking became clearer but it was not until 1950 when Richard Doll and A.B. Hill published the key paper in the *British Medical Journal*[11] that the evidence was sufficient to make the link between smoking and lung cancer. The 'Counterblaste against Tobacco' by King James VI has already been mentioned.

In *Rob Roy* by Sir Walter Scott, an occasional pipe and tobacco are called for, to leave the person with both to meditate and have some peace. Scott then uses a quotation from an old song:

> The Indian leaf doth briefly burn;
> So doth man's strength to weakness turn;—
> The fire of youth extinguished quite,
> Comes age, like embers, dry and white
> Think of this as you take tobacco.

Here is an early warning of the dangers of tobacco.

In a short book entitled *Poems and parodies in praise of tobacco (An odd volume for smokers. A Lyttlel Parcel of Poems and Parodies in praise of Tobacco Collected by Walter Hamilton)* there are 180 pages of poems, mainly in relation to pipe smoking, though some to cigarettes.[12] Only a few are of Scottish origin. This short anonymous one matches the verse from Scott:

> The Cigarette (no date)
> I am only a small cigarette
> But my work I will get in, you bet
>   For the stern coffin maker
>   And the grim undertaker,
> Will declare I bring fish to their net.[13]

This sets out the employment consequences which follow from smoking; it's a profitable job to be an undertaker.

There is an interesting poem on 'My Best Pipe' which was published in the University News Sheet from St Andrews, March 1886:

> **Ballade of the Best Pipe.**
> I hear you fervently extol
>   The virtues of your ancient clay
> As black as any piece of coal
> To me it smells of rank decay

242

And bones of people passed away
   A smell I never could admire
With all respect to you I say
   Give me a finely seasoned briar.

. . .

   Envoy
Clay, meerschaum, hookah, what are they
   That I should view them with desire
I'll sing till all my hair is grey
   Give me a finely seasoned briar.[14]

This next poem comes from *A pedlar's Pack of Ballads and songs* (1869).[15] It runs:

The Cutty

When nobs come oot to walk aboot
And show their shapes to leddies
They're ne'er withoot their grand cheroot
For that they think well bread is

And when they meet-no in the street
But ablins ower a meal like –
Then oot they draw a meerschaum braw
An' that looks real genteel like.

Weel! There's nae ban on ony man
Let him be braw or sootie
I'll no debar their grand cigar
But I'll haud to my cutty.

The 'Cutty' is a short pipe, often locally made, Stonehaven being an important source.

Finally, Lord Byron writes on tobacco from his poem 'The Island':

. . . Sublime tobacco . . .
Magnificent in Stamboul, but less grand
But not less loved, in Wapping or the Strand;
Divine in hookahs, glorious in a pipe
When tipped with amber, mellow, rich, and ripe;
Like other charmers, wooing the caress
More dazzlingly when daring in full dress
Yet thy true lovers more admire by far
Thy naked beauties, – give me a cigar![16]

What matters most to the Gentleman is his cigar.

Poverty and industrialisation

'Poverty Parts Good Company', Joanna Baillie (1762–1851)

Joanna Baillie spent her girlhood in Glasgow and went to school there. Her father was a Dr Baillie who became professor of Divinity in Glasgow. He died two years after his appointment and the family went to live in Long Calderwood, Joanna's mother being a sister of William and John Hunter. When John died he left his collections in London to Matthew Baillie, Joanna's brother. His collection was given to the Royal College of Surgeons in London and Joanna's family then moved to London, and lived in Great Windmill Street with her brother. The Hunter brothers were the dominant medical teachers in London in the 18th century. William Hunter's collection came to the University of Glasgow and established the Hunterian Museum. The poem records the problem of becoming poor and the effect this has in relationships:

'Poverty Parts Good Company'
When my o'erlay was white as the foam o' the linn,
And siller was clinking my pouches within,
When my lambkins were bleating on meadow and brae
As I went to my love in new cleeding say gay,
Kind was she, and my friends were free;
But poverty parts good company.

> We met at the fair, and we met at the kirk;
> We met i' the sunshine, we met in the mirk;
> And the sound of her voice and the blinks o' her een
> The cheering and life of my bosom ha'e been.
> The leaves frae the tree at Martinmas flee,
> And poverty parts sweet company
>
> But the hope o' my love is a cure for its smart
> And the spaewife has tald me to keep up my heart;
> For wi' my last saxpence her loof I ha'e crossed
> And the bliss that is fated can never be lost
> Though cruelly we may ilka day see
> Our poverty parts dear company.'[17]

His whole life broken by poverty and his dream vanished.

'Effie: A Ballad', Janet Hamilton (1795–1873)

Janet Hamilton was born in the parish of Shotts but moved to Old Monklands in Lanarkshire where she remained for the rest of her life. She learned to read as a child and used the village library where she read widely. She wrote prolifically. During the last eighteen years of her life, when she was blind, her husband read to her and her son was her amanuensis. She was a strong advocate of temperance.

The ballad begins in sadness:

> She was wearin' awa! She was wearin' awa!
> Wi' the leaves of October we thocht she would fa';
> For her cheeks were ower red, and her e'e was owre bricht
> Where the saul leukit out like an angel of licht.[18]
>
> The auldest of five, when a lassie of ten
> She had baith the house and the bairnies to fen';
> The mither was gane when she was a bairn
> Sae Effie had mony sad lessons to learn

But she tries, she's kind and she and looked after her brothers and sisters. When she reaches her teens she falls in love with Jamie, they woo, and he promises to love her for ever. Then her father comes home from church one winter's morning and announces that the wedding banns have been read between Jamie and Katie MacLean. Kate has an inheritance which Jamie considers more attractive than Effie. She is devastated, and her lip quivers, but 'nae word could she speak'. She has done her best but her whole life:

> Was silently meltin' awa.' And by October,
> An' sae she was wearin' fast wearin' awa,
> Wi' the leaves of October sweet Effie did fa'.
> Her mournin' was ended, an blissfu' and bricht
> The dear lassie dwells wi' the angels o' licht.

Thus ends this tragic story of a young woman who brings up the family from the age of ten, but loses out because she is poor, and dies of a broken heart.

The development of heavy industry is well set up in this next poem.

From a Ballad in Blank Verse, Greenock.
John Davidson. (1857–1909)

The villages that sleep the winter through
And waken with the spring, keep festival
All summer and Autumn: this grey town
That pipes the morning up before the lark
With shrieking steam, and from a hundred stalks
Lacquers the sooty sky; where hammers clang
On iron hulls, and cranes in harbours creak
Rattle and swing. Whole cargoes on their necks
Where men sweat gold that others hoard or spend,
And lurk like vermin in their narrow streets:
This grey old town, this firth, the further strand
Spangled with hamlets, and the wooded steeps,. . .[19]

The dirt and the noise are here graphically described in one of Scotland's growing industrial towns. There is, in addition the comment that while some sweat, others make money at their expense.

'The Last Sark', Ellen Johnston (1835–1873)

Johnston was born in Hamilton and she published a series of poems under the pseudonym of 'Factory girl'. She died destitute in the Barony Poorhouse in Glasgow.

'The Last Sark'

Gude guide me, are ye hame again, and hae ye got nae wark?
We've nothing noo tae pit awa, unless your auld blue shirt [pawn]
My heid is rinnin' roon aboot, far lichter than a flee
What care some gentry if they're weel though a' the puir wad dee?

Our merchants and mill-masters they wad never want a meal
Though a' the banks in Scotland was for a twalmonth fail
For some o them hae far mair gowd than ony ane can see
What care some gentry if they're weel though a' the puir wad dee?

Our hoose aince bien and cosy, John, oor beds aince snug and warm,
Feels unco cauld and dismal noo, and empty as a barn
The weans sit greetin in our face, and we hae nocht to gie
What care some gentry if they're weel though a' the puir wad dee?

It is the puir man's hard-won cash that fills the rich man's purse;
I'm sure his gowden coffers they are het wi mony a curse
Were it no for the workin man what wad the rich man be?
What care some gentry if they're weel though a' the puir wad dee?

My head is licht, my heart is weak, my een and growing blin';
The bair is fa'en aff my knee – oh! John catch haud o' him
You ken I hinna tasted meat for days far mair than three:
Were it no for my helpless bairns I wadna care to dee.[20]

A depressing tale of a woman run off her feet, exhausted, who has had no real food for days, and she even drops her baby off her knee. Death again, if it was not for her children, would be a comfort.

'St Rollox Lum's Address to its Brethren'(1842), John Mitchell

This poem sets out what Glasgow looks like from the top of a tall chimney in the St Rollox steel factory in the north of the city. Mitchell was born in Paisley. The poem begins:

> Haud up your heads, ye stunted things
> Or gudesake get the len o' wings
> And soar aloft like me, where sings
> The cheery lark
> When frae its dewy bed it springs
> In some green park
>
> I see that frae the morning's dawn
> Till ev'ning has her curtain drawn
> Ye spread your vapours o'er the lan'
> Sae thick, in faith
> That those who pass you aft maun stan'
> An' gasp for breath[21]

The smell, the smoke and the breathing problems are clear, and there is a suggestion that the people below are stunted with growth problems. An issue well recognised in the city, and associated also with rickets.

'System', Robert Louis Stevenson

This short poem, with a strange title, appears in *A Child's Garden of Verse* (1885) and is relevant to discussions on the issues of poverty.[22] It is a reflection of Stevenson's own upbringing in the New Town in Edinburgh, not far from the tenements of the city's poor housing. The poem highlights the difference between the rich and the poor child:

> Every night my prayers I say,
> And get my dinner every day;
> And every day that I've been good,
> I get an orange after food.

The child that is not clean and neat,
With lots of toys and things to eat,
He is a naughty child I'm sure
Or else his dear papa is poor.

Around twenty years before this was written, there was a major public health problem in Edinburgh which is highlighted nicely in this poem and which was mentioned in the introduction to this book, when a tenement in the High Street collapsed and thirty-five people were killed and many others wounded. During the rescue operations, a voice was heard to cry 'Heave awa lads, I'm no deid yet' and a boy was pulled from the rubble. This is commemorated in Paisley's Close in the High Street with those words carved above the entrance. Following this Dr Henry Duncan Littlejohn was appointed Medical Officer of Health. Stevenson must have been aware of the health issues and poverty in the city and this poem is reminder of the two classes who lived in Edinburgh, and the differences between the old city and the New Town.

The quality of water

For many reasons, clean water is an essential requirement for any community. Until the middle of the 19th century water was generally available from pumps, steams or rivers. The quality varied enormously and there were frequent episodes of infection, notably cholera. Public health measures were limited, though the most famous of these was in London where Dr John Snow in 1855, who recognised the infection problem in a pump in Soho, and removed the handle of the pump. The first two of these poems recognise the dangers of the water in Glasgow, and the third hails the real change, the clean waters of Loch Katrine which were pumped to Glasgow and opened by Queen Victoria in 1859 as a major public health triumph. In this poem the unpleasant aspects of the Clyde are set out:

'Ode to the Clyde' (1910), Charles J. Kirk
Hail great black-bosomed mother of our city
Whose odoriferous breath offends the earth
Whose cats and dogs excite our pity
As they sail past with aldermanic girth

No salmon hast thou in jet black waters
Save what is adhering to the tins
Thus thy adorers-Govan's lovely daughters —
adorn thy shrine with offerings for their sins.

Yet thou art great. Though strangers hold their noses
When sailing down to Rothesay at the fair
Thy exiled sons would barter tons of roses
To scent thy sweetness on the desert air.[23]

Here then is a picture of the Clyde with dead and bloated animals and a terrible smell, yet still loved by Glaswegians.

'Wanted in Glasgow' (1876), Marion Bernstein

This second poem empasises the lethal nature of the water.

Wanted a filter to filter the Clyde
After some hundreds of people have died,
Chancing to fall in its poisonous tide;
Those who fall in there are likely to bide,
If they have opened their mouths very wide
They may as well stay, for when dragged out and dried
'Twill be found that although they're not drowned thay have died
Merely by trying the taste of the Clyde.[24]

'A Welcome to the Waters of Loch Katrine' (1863), James Nicholson

Nicholson was born in Edinburgh in 1822 and came to Glasgow to work as a tailor in the Govan Workhouse. He learned to read, and his first poem was published when he was nineteen years old. He published in various magazines and a thin volume was printed in 1850. Before he died in 1897 the Govan Parochial Board presented the poet with an address in which his long and faithful services were recognised. The poem describes the value of clean water:

'A Welcome to the Waters of Loch Katrine'

Thou comest to a city where men ultimately die,

Where hearts in grief are swelling, and cheeks are seldom dry

A city where merchant princes to Mammon basely kneel

While those who drag the idol's car are crushed beneath the wheel.

Throughout her might system of tunnel and tube and main,

They healthful current is pulsing, pulsing through every vein;

In the fever den, in the attic, in cellars under the street,

The poor have long been waiting to quaff thy waters sweet.

Thou comest in thy beauty, like Godiva, long ago,

To save our sin-cursed city from a tax of death and woe

To cool the fire of fever, and quench the fever of lust

To moisten the lips of the dying, and moisten the poor man's crust.

O would thy gushing waters might quench for ever and aye

Those fountains of fiery ruin that lead men's souls astray;

That drunkeries were all abolished, and , planted in their stead

The reading room and the school room, and shops for the sale of bread![25]

This poem records the great achievement of the Loch Katrine Scheme. Cholera was still rife in Scotland and there had been epidemics in 1837, 1848 and 1853. Cholera returned in 1865-6 when only fifty-three people died compared to an earlier epidemic in which 4,000 died.[26] This was a very significant improvement in health achieved by bringing clean water to the city.

An end piece

Willie Winkie, William Miller (1810–1872)

William Miller has been said to have written the greatest nursery song in the world; there is a monument set up to him in the Glasgow Necropolis. He was born in the Briggate in Glasgow but spent his early life in Parkhead, a village in the east end. He had intended being a surgeon, but a severe illness forced him to stop his studies and he became a wood turner. He contributed articles to many periodicals. This poem is included here as an example of family life and a little boy who doesn't get much sleep, and neither do his parents. However, it is noted that a 'kiss frae aff his rosie lips gives strength anew to me.'; a suitable ending to a chapter on social issues and health.

Willie Winkie

Wee Willie Winkie rins through the toun,
Up stairs and doun stairs in his nicht goun,
Tirlin' at the windon, crying at the lock,
Are the weans in their bed, for it's now ten o'clock?

Hey, Willie Winkie, are ye comin' ben?
The cat's singin' grey thrums to the sleepin' hen
The dog's speldert on the floor, and doesna gie a cheep
But here's a waurife laddie that fa' asleep.

Onything but sleep, you rogue, glowerin' like the moon,
Rattlin' in an airn jug wi' an airn spoon [iron]
Rumblin', tumblin', roun' about, crawin' like a cock,
Skirlin' like a kenna-what, waukenin' sleepin' folk.

Hey Willie Winkie, the wean's in a creel
Wamblin' aff a body's knee like a very eel
Ruggin' at the cat's lug, and ravelin' a' her thrums
Hey Willie Winkie-see there he comes.

Wearied is the mither that has a stourie wean, [rushing about]
A wee stumpie stousie that canna rin his lane, [plump child]
That has a battle aye wi' sleep before he'll close an e'e,
But a kiss frae aff his rosie lips gies strength anew to me.[27]

Conclusions

It was noted at the start of this chapter that there were few references to poverty and social conditions in the mainstream literature. This is surprising in view of the evidence and the contemporary writings and images which were widely available. For example, reference has already been made to the writings of Thomas Chalmers, but add to this the work of the Medical Officers of Health (Sir Henry Littlejohn in Edinburgh and Dr J.B. Russell in Glasgow) and the additional information provided by early photographers such as Thomas Annan and Hill and Adamson. Chalmers' work sets out in a most vivid way the living conditions in cities such as Glasgow with slums and tenements. In addition it is strange that there are no contemporary detective stories set in Scotland. Such a genre provides a way to document the seamier side of life and living conditions. The earliest detective mystery is generally regarded as *Murders in the Rue Morgue* (1841) by Edward Allen Poe, but the most famous was Sir Arthur Connan Doyle's *Sherlock Holmes*. The main character, Sherlock Holmes, was based on Dr Joseph Bell one of Doyle's teacher's in the medical school in Edinburgh. In addition there is no work in the 19th century which refers to the goings on of the resurrectionists, (the Sack 'em up men), Burke and Hare and Dr Robert Knox the anatomist. This had to wait until the 20th century to be described in the literature of Scotland.

With all of this evidence available why is there such a gap when writers in England and elsewhere tell powerful stories about poverty and health? The most likely reason is Victorian sensibility in Scotland coupled with a strong Presbyterian ethos. Why, in the expansion of the merchant class in cities such as Glasgow would the emerging middle class wish to read about or view poverty and poor living conditions? The rise of the labour movement, chartism, and indeed communism, which made it possible to describe and discuss such issues came at the end of the century. Thomas Johnston's Book *The History of the Working Classes in Scotland* describes these changes in detail.[28] This may not explain entirely the reasons why there is a paucity in the literature of such subjects, and more research remains to be done.

Notes

1   Chalmers, *Health of Glasgow*, p. 2.

2   Thomas Chalmers, *Problems of Poverty: An Enquiry into the Industrial Condition of the Poor* (London: Thomas Nelson and Sons, 1912).

3   John Mayne, 'Glasgow', in *Mungo's Tongues: Glasgow Poems 1630–1990*, ed. Hamish Whyte (Edinburgh: Mainstream Publishing, 1993), pp. 33–6.

4   Anonymous, 'How We Spent the Sabbath Day', in Whyte, *Mungo's Tongues*, p. 104–11, ll. 1–7.

5   John Galt, *The Provost* (Oxford: Oxford University Press, 1982).

6   Margaret Oliphant, *Passages in the Life of Mrs Margaret Maitland of Sunnyside, Written by Herself* (New York: D. Appleton, 1851).

7   J. M. Barrie, *Auld Licht Idylls* (London: Hodder and Stoughton, 1934).

8   'The Demon Drink', in McGonagall, *Last Poetic Gems*, pp. 11–13.

9   James P. Crawford, 'The Drunkard's Raggit Wean', in George Eyre-Todd, *The Glasgow Poets: Their Lives and Poems* (Glasgow and Edinburgh: William Hodge and Company, 1903), pp. 632–3.

10   Janet Hamilton, 'Oor Location', in Crawford & Imlah, *New Penguin Scottish Verse*, pp. 342–3, ll. 1–38.

11   Richard Doll and A.B. Hill, 'Smoking and Carcinoma of the Lung', *British Medical Journal* (2), pp. 739–48.

12   Walter Hamilton, ed., *Poems and Parodies in Praise of Tobacco (An Odd Volume for Smokers: A Lyttlel Parcel of Poems and Parodies in Praise of Tobacco Collected by Walter Hamilton)*, (London: Reeves and Turner, 1889).

13   Ibid., p. 89.

14   Ibid, Anonymous, 'Ballade of the Best Pipe', pp. 174–5, ll. 1–8 and ll. 125–128.

15   W.H. Logan, 'The Cutty', in *A Pedlar's Pack of Ballads and Songs* (Edinburgh: W. Paterson, 1869), pp. 58–9.

16   Lord Byron, 'The Island', in Hamilton, *Poems and Parodies in Praise of Tobacco*, p. 32, l. 11 and ll. 15–22.

17   Joanna Baillie, 'Poverty Parts Good Company', in Eyre-Todd, *The Glasgow Poets*, pp. 97–9.

18   Janet Hamilton, 'Effie: A Ballad', in Eyre-Todd, *The Glasgow Poets*, p. 228–232, ll. 1–4.

19   John Davidson, 'Greenock: From a Ballad in Blank Verse', in *A Book of Scottish Verse*, ed. E.L. Mackie (Oxford: Oxford University Press, 1956), p. 385.

20   Ellen Johnston, 'The Last Sark', in Crawford & Imlah, *New Penguin Book of Verse*, p. 366.

21   John Mitchell, 'St Rollox Lum's Address to its Brethren', in Whyte, *Mungo's Tongues*, pp. 96–102, ll. 1–6 and ll. 13–18.

22   Robert Louis Stevenson, 'System', in *A Child's Garden of Verse* (London: Longmans Green and Co., 1926), p. 20.

23   Charles J. Kirk, 'Ode to the Clyde', in Whyte, *Mungo's Tongues*, p. 156.

24   Marion Bernstein, 'Wanted in Glasgow', in Whyte, *Mungo's Tongues*, pp. 141–2, ll. 1–8.

25   James Nicholson, 'A Welcome to the Waters of Loch Katrine', in Whyte, *Mungo's Tongues*, pp. 131–2.

26   T.C. Smout, *A Century of the Scottish People 1830–1950* (London: Fontana Press, 1986), p. 43.

27   William Miller, 'Willie Winkie', in Eyre-Todd, *The Glasgow Poets*, pp. 302–3.

28   Johnston, *History of the Working Classes*.

CHAPTER 16

Learning from literature

Give me ae spark o' natures fire
That's a' the learning I desire.
Robert Burns

The quote from Burns' 'The Epistle to John Lapraik' sets the scene for this chapter. How do doctors and the health-care team learn about the complexity of modern clinical practice, when it changes almost daily? In the midst of the evidence and the increasing knowledge base, how does the clinical team retain its humanity? In addition how do patients and the public keep up with these advances and remain involved in their care, and in the wider public health implications of new knowledge?

Apart from the obvious literary, historical and medical aspects of this book, there is a broader purpose, identified in the introduction, of providing resources for medical practitioners and other clinical professions to reflect on what they do in everyday clinincal practice. Extracts from poetry and prose have illustrated the power of literature, and the sensitivity of the author to describe a range of health-related matters. Many have also commented on the role of the doctor in society, as a teacher and as an advocate for the patient. There are also messages for patients and the public to consider their lifestyles, environment and the social circumstances of their health. There are messages too for politicians.

The extracts have illustrated the determinants of health in a very vivid way, and from such readings it is not difficult to see how the health of Scotland's population has been influenced, with diet, alcohol and poverty being some of the many issues which were raised. In addition, the complexity of clinical practice has been made clear in relation to the ethical issues debated, and the difficulties in making clinical decisions. The importance of effective analysis of the problem and the role of judgement in coming

256

to a conclusion, have also been described. More importantly perhaps, is the way in which patients have, or have not, been involved in the decision making process. This process is likely to continue to be important, as more complex, expensive and effective treatments become available, as medical science continues to open up new areas for research, and as patients become more sophisticated and have greater access to information through the internet. The issues of risk and uncertainty in determining the most effective outcome will remain. The extracts are meant to stimulate the reader (professional, patient or a member of the public) to think about the subject, and for that reason my analysis has been deliberately limited to the explanation of some of the language and of clinical facts.

For clinical staff the keeping of a commonplace book of papers, thoughts, ideas which have been of help, may be useful. If commonplace books have any place they should also be for patients and carers to develop themselves or to use with others for understanding and support.

Most of the readings in this chapter come from the 20th or 21st centuries, periods of enormous change in medicine, in almost every area of clinical practice and public health. There is now much greater understanding of the biological aspects of how the body functions through the work on genetics and the role of DNA in illness. New treatments and diagnostic investigations have been established and new diseases have been identified such as HIV infection. The skill base of the doctor has been expanded enormously and requires continual updating. Teamwork is now a key part of clinical care.

One of the important issues raised, indirectly, has been the provision of a health service and how it is funded. The 19th century perspective has been particularly relevant as new procedures and treatments were developed, including vaccination, but which, for those in rural areas and those who could not afford such procedures, were unavailable. It is easy to overlook the enormous benefits of a national health service.

Some of the selections which have been used also allow personal considerations on health and illness. They raise questions such as:

If it was me, what would I do?
What if it was my mother or child?

257

Would I have the courage to tackle societal problems such as poverty or alcohol addiction?

Could I become an advocate for health?

These readings also raise the importance of emotions, and getting involved in the care of patients. The need for empathy, compassion and the value of communication challenges the old assumption that doctors should not become emotionally involved with patients.

The texts quoted and referred to all emphasise the importance of learning and not only updating medical knowledge, but re-thinking one's own personal approach to health and illness in relation to the patient in front of you. The need, and ability, to change thinking and practice will continue to be vital as new procedures, therapies and diagnostic techniques are developed. The role of the arts and humanities in clinical education also become clearer, with involvement of students (and as they go on to become members of one of the clinical professions) with real practical experience in one or more of the arts.

For me, this involvement in the arts has been especially important. In particular, literature has stimulated a re-thinking of clinical practice, and highlighted how communication and care are set right at the heart of the patient-doctor relationship.

Approaching the opportunities

At its simplest, an anthology from the literature of Scotland, or a common-place book of ideas and thoughts, can provide the foundation of a learning resource; a series of texts which have general relevance to health, illness and the role of the doctor. I have deliberately limited my commentary on the texts as their potential impact rests with the reader and not with the interpreter. In this way, over the centuries, one can follow the development of clinical science, the role of the doctor, the development of health services, and the ethical issues involved.

In addition to this there is a need to consider the context and settings for learning in medicine and the other clinical professions. Learning can occur in lectures, tutorials, small group teaching, laboratories, bedside teaching and in the community. Sir William Osler's comment at the beginning of this book that literature was to bring the author and the reader 'mind to mind' is very relevant. Much of the learning involves the listening to, and the telling of stories, and the role of the narrative of medicine is now widely recognised.[1] As the 20th century progressed, film, television and magazines rapidly developed the taste for medical dramas, which provided, for some, the impetus to take up medicine as a profession. Some of the earliest of these were the *Doctor in the House* stories by Richard Gordon in 1952, followed by the film version in 1954. The character Simon Sparrow is a hapless medical student and Sir Lancelot Spratt, a distinguished surgeon. *Dr Finlay's Case Book,* based on the writings of A.J. Cronin, was another example of this. In veterinary medicine there was a similar boost to the profession by the stories of James Herriot (Alf Wright) whose first book *If Only They Could Talk* (1970) led to a series of others. Within this context therefore the written word, used singly or in groups, can provide the same stimulus for learning, hence the importance of having such appropriate material, this being one of the objectives of this book.

It is also relevant to consider the potential for patients and their families to assess such writings. In reading groups, counselling groups and in creative writing sessions there are opportunities for all to find inspiration and encouragement. Personal experience as a doctor practising in the cancer area suggests strongly that patients are not only highly sophisticated but can contribute in a very positive way to the discussion. The professionals can learn from patients, indeed one of my most powerful learning experiences was in listening to cancer patients and their families share their thoughts on the care provided.

There are a number of issues which flow from this approach: understanding changes in clinical practice, defining the determinants of health, outlining the role and competence of the doctor, capturing the patient perspective and the development of the curriculum. The range of literature covered here is necessarily restricted because of space, and the reader is asked to identify other examples from personal reading and add to this resource.

Understanding changes in clinical practice

The first issue is an appreciation of the change, progression and improvements in health and medical care over time. It becomes a fascinating history of health and medicine told through pens of storytellers and poets, who have illustrated the changes which have occurred. A few additional brief extracts have been chosen to illustrate this change and these have been chosen mainly from 20th and 21st century Scottish literature.

Health services

The problem of infection has always been a serious one. In *The Silver Darlings* by Neil Gunn (1891–1973), Finn walks many miles to find a doctor because of what he calls the plague.[2] It is likely that this was around 1832. He arrives in Wick to meet the doctor having walked for two days without food or drink. The doctor receives him kindly, indeed he is introduced to a specialist who has come from the city to help with the problem, probably cholera. He is given a prescription, treated with great kindliness, given some food and sent on his way; this emphasises the problem of being cared for without a health service.

The development of hospitals is a major topic on its own. This poem in *Random Rhymes,* written just before the NHS began to celebrate a 'Castle of Healing', refers to the Western Infirmary in Glasgow:

> A mighty castle rears its walls,
> Upon the banks of Kelvin stream,
> And hundreds throng within its hall,
> And lights from myriad windows gleam.
> The knights within can wield their steel
> With skill the ancients could not gain,
> And monsters grim they bring to heel,
> The dragons of disease and pain.

No shrinking maids, the ladies there,
They face life's troubles with a will,
Real heroines who do and dare
They tend and sooth with gentle skill.
The gates have seen the inward flow
Of ill and helpless carried through,
And thousand too who outward go,
Restored in health to start anew.[3]

It is concerned not only with the medical staff, the 'Knights', but with the outcome of care, and in particular the role of the nursing staff, the real heroines.

Medical students

'The White-Maa's saga' by Eric Linklater (1929), is an early story about medical students and their trial and tribulations.[4] Linklater had himself been a medical student in Aberdeen, but had given it up for writing. A White-Maa is a herring-gull, and is the nickname for the main character in the book, Peter Flett. An Orcadian, he is a medical student at the University of Inverdoon, readily identified as Aberdeen. It begins with him the failing the 2nd MB exam, a common occurrence as many of the students have, just a few years before, returned from fighting in the First World War. Alcohol excess often followed such events and these episodes are related realistically. While the students do maternity training they stay in the Howdie Digs and wait to take part in deliveries. As Peter starts his study for his re-sits the following is observed:

That had decided Peter, and he had started the study of medicine with an enthusiasm which carried him through his first year. But in his second year enthusiasm began to get leg-weary and think of sitting on benches and unbuttoning after noon. For the scientific acquisition of knowledge is almost as tedious as the routine acquisition of wealth. The medical student's education is full of interest – it is even exciting – to the casual observer. But steadfastly for five years to commit to memory the minute details of

261

even the most exciting facts requires a prodigious mental effort and almost inevitably connotes boredom. A well-dissected arm is a pretty sight, and the story of the endocrine glands is as absorbing as a mystery novel with the last chapter torn away.

Linklater's narrator also comments on student life:

> There is almost unlimited freedom in the extra-collegiate life of the Scots University. There are no residential colleges, no university discipline beyond the lecture room. Students live in lodgings of their own selection.

Having gone home to Orkney for a while he returns again to Inverdoon to try once more. In the bar one evening Peter and his friends get taking about 'civilization' and there is an interesting medical twist to the discussion. The students are discussing world issues:

> Civilization connotes change certainly, but not necessarily superiority. It means factories instead of pasture land, tram-cars instead of walking, complicated interdependence instead of independence. Civilization means that we invent cures for diseases which naturally tend to disappear. . . and evolve new diseases for which there is no remedy. Personally I always spell it 'syphilization'.

Peter also considers how he will make a living:

> It wasn't a case of making only his living. It was a case of making his life, and he couldn't make his life in an office. Medicine was a better profession than most, for you dealt with people, no ledgers or law books or dusty files; but the way to it was three years long, three years of printed words, and the stimulus of completion was too far off to carry him.

Some in the early 21st century might consider that the ledgers and law books are what medicine has become. He fails the exam a third time, romantic alliances intrude, and there is an unexpected ending. The ethos of the medical student and the problems and aspirations are well described.

Developments in science

Poor Things by Alasdair Gray develops a theme which raised hackles in Glasgow in the early 1800s.[5] Namely, the re-animation of corpses by Glasgow anatomists, tried out on criminals who had been hanged. Here Gray (and it is a complex story) has a corpse of a young woman resuscitated after she has drowned. The twist is that she is also pregnant and the baby is alive so the brain is also transplanted.

The Wasp Factory[6] by Ian Banks is a remarkable story of science and medicine and its manipulation. It is complex with a fascinating denouement which the reader will have to find out on their own and consider the implications.

The way we think about research, the future and what it might mean to us is brilliantly noted in a short poem by Jimmy Black as he considers it:

Real Life
Transmit this advice, Lord, tae aw would be weans
Who hope soon to sample this earth's joys and pains
Direct them to shun scientific creators
Who tinker wi' test tubes and strange incubators
When intae this life you've a notion for comin'
Just try to make sure that your maw is a wumman[7]

James Bridie (O H Mavor, 1888–1951), one of the most interesting playwrights of the 20th century was, of course, a doctor. His play *The Sleeping Clergyman* (1934) takes us through the story of a family and their relationships.[8] Within that family there is a series of doctors, one of whom eventually discovers the cure for a major pandemic. It describes the importance of research, the arrogance of doctors, their compassion for individuals and the public and shows some of the complexity of being a clinician, on the one hand wishing to push forward research and improve care, and on the other a willingness and a need to look after the individual.

The story begins with conflict between Cameron, an untidy young man dying of tuberculosis, but interested in medical research, and Marshall the established doctor.

Cameron: Have you ever heard of Pasteur

Marshall: No. Yes. The French chemist

Cameron: Do you know his work on ferments?

Marshall: What? . . . Oh, yes, he believes in spontaneous generation, doesn't he?

Cameron: Oh my God, Spallanzani killed that a hundred years ago. Do you never read your Voltaire?

Marshall: Voltaire was not a man of Science

Cameron: And you are I suppose? And you don't know what Pasteur is doing. Neither does he for that matter. But you know what Joe Lister's doing?

Marshall: Yes. Poisoning his patients with carbolic. And why? Because of germs, ha ha. Because of germs he pretends to see floating in the air. Lister's a fine fellow, but that kind of thing isn't far removed from delusional insanity. . .

Marshall: Look here young Cameron, you stick to facts. Our profession has been storing facts since the days of Hippocrates, and they are good enough for me and good enough for you. You leave Lister to people the circumambient ether with infusorial animalcula.

Soon after, Cameron dies, having married, and leaves his wife to deliver twins, a boy and a girl, then she dies. The boy moves into medicine and eventually becomes the person who develops a successful vaccine against a new virus, as dangerous as the pandemic flu which has just passed over. The clinical trial is carried out, and is a success.

Curiosity and discovery

The extract above leads into a discussion of the subjects of curiosity and discovery, important components of the role of the doctor. Acting as a 'medical detective' the doctor has an obligation not only to find out the cause of the signs and symptoms in a particular patient but to have a role more generally in improving health and treating illness. The curiosity is important: many medical discoveries have happened because of a chance observation, the discovery of penicillin by Alexander Fleming being a classic example. Instilling the trait of curiosity is not simply about mastering the facts, figures and skills which are learned in medical school. It concerns the way clinical practice is carried out. Always looking and searching for something new or different can give a clue to better diagnosis or treatment. It is being a medical detective; able to find clues, to investigate and come up with novel solutions. Robert Burns in his 'Epistle to John Lapraik' quoted at the head of this chapter, sets out his views when he criticizes schools and colleges, for confusing student's brains. His answer is clear;

> Give me ae spark o' Natures fire
> That's a' the learning I desire.[9]

It is more than just learning, it is a way of thinking and responding to problems. It is a key attribute of the doctor.

Specialisation

This has been one of the continuing features of modern medicine over the last hundred years. The medical profession has moved from being a profession of generalists to one of specialists with the general practitioner (family practitioner) remaining the generalist – and even that is changing. This has important implications for the delivery of care, the quality of care provided and the way in which doctors keep up to date and regularly review their own performance.

Disability

Disability is a neglected subject, as are the feelings and attitudes to such problems. In Robin Jenkin's book *The Cone-Gatherers* (2004) he sets out some of the issues.[10] This extract occurs early in the book where he discusses two disabled people who live in a hut and pick the cones in the wood for a living:

> They peeled their potatoes the night before and left them in a pot of cold water. They did not wash before they started to eat or cook. They did not change their clothes. They had no table; an upturned box instead, with a newspaper for a cloth and each sat on his own bed. They seldom spoke.

All evening they would be dumb, the taller brooding over a days old paper, the dwarf carving some animal out of wood; at present he was making a squirrel. Seeing it half-finished that afternoon, holding it shudderingly in his hands, Duror had against his will, indeed against the whole frenzied thrust of his being, sensed the kinship between the carver and the creature whose likeness he was carving. When complete, the squirrel would be not only recognizable, it would be almost alive. To Duror it had been the final defeat that such ability should be in a half-man, a freak, an imbecile. He had read that the Germans were putting idiots and cripples to death in gas chambers. Outwardly, as everybody expected, he condemned such barbarity; inwardly, thinking of idiocy and crippledness not as abstraction but as embodied in the crouchbacked cone-gatherer, he profoundly approved.

Hugh MacDiarmid adds an interesting comment on disability and the way in which others see those affected in his poem 'In the Children's Hospital', [11]

Does it matter-losing your legs?. . . Siegfried Sassoon

Now let the legless boy show the great lady
How well he can manage his crutches.
It doesn't matter though the Sister objects,
'He's not used to them yet' when such is
The will of the Princess. Come, Tommy,
Try a few desparate steps through the ward.
Then the hand of Royalty will pat your head
And life will suddenly cease to be hard.
For a couple of legs are surely no miss
When the loss leads to such an honour as this!
One knows, when one sees how jealous the rest
Of the children are, it's been all for the best! –
But would the sound of your sticks on the floor
Thunder in her skull for evermore!

This gives an interesting insight into the feelings of those who are disabled and on the perceptions of others.

Patient perspectives on science and medicine

As is proper, patients and their families know more and more about illness and its treatment, and in the ways in which disease can be prevented. The following four extracts show this clearly.

'Cholesterol'

This song by Adam McNaughton illustrates the knowledge, but not necessarily the willingness, to change. It was in response to a 'Good Hearted Glasgow' campaign, an initiative to improve the health of the people of Glasgow. Although the message has been heard and understood, behavioural change is limited!

> I've been taking advice on the right things to eat
> Since shortly before I was born
> Frae the national dried milk and the cod liver oil
> Tae powdered rhinoceros horn
> In they days they'd tell us tae lay aff the starches
> The sugar, potatoes and breid
> Now they've done a U-turn, tell us the breid and potatoes
> Will give us the fibre we need.
>
> So I've made up my mind that the menus designed
> By the experts just arenae for me
> Nae trained dietician or general practitioner
> Dictate what I'll have for my tea
> Brown bread with the low fat paste thinly spread on
> May be healthier than a meat pie
> By who wants to grow old eating St Ivel Gold
> I would rather taste butter and die
>
> Cholesterol, cholesterol
> My chance of surviving is small
> But I'll no get a does o' anorexia nervosa
> 'Cause I love my cholesterol.

267

But I'm no gonnae take the suggestions they make
About changing the way that I eat
Cutting oot cheese and nae chips if you please,
nae chocolate, nae ice cream, nae meat
they tell you to give up these goodies below
and they promise you pie in the sky
well semi-skimmed milk might diminish my bulk
but I'll take double cream till I die.

Cholesterol, cholesterol
My chance of surviving is small
The way that I dine I'm on course for angina
But I love my cholesterol.[12]

The second two poems come from two of Scotland's greatest contemporary
authors. Both died of cancer.

'Gorgo and Beau'

This poem, from Edwin Morgan compares two cells; Gorgo, a cancer cell,
and Beau, a normal cell. Gorgo, the cancer cell begins:

GORGO: My old friend Beau, we meet again. How goes it?
Howzit gaun? Wie geht's? Ca va? Eh?
BEAU: Same old Gorgo, flashing your credentials:
Any time, any place, any tongue, and race, you are there.
It is bad enough doing what you do,
But to boast about it – why do I talk to you?
GORGO: You talk to me because you find it interesting
I am different. I stimulate the brain matter
Your mates are virtual clones –
BEAU: – oh rubbish –
GORGO: you know what I mean. Your paths are laid down.
Your functions are clear. Your moves are gentlemanly
You even know when to die gracefully.
Nothing is more boring than a well-made body.

Why should this be? That's what you don't know.
And that is why you talk to me.

. . .

BEAU: you think you can overturn pain with a cartoon?
GORGO: Pain, what is pain, I have never felt it
Though I have watched our human hosts give signs –
A gasp, a groan, a spasm, a scream-whatever it is. . . . .
BEAU: shall I tell you about suffering?
Imagine a male cancer ward; morning;
Curtains are swished back, urine bottles emptied,
Medications laid out. 'Another day, another dollar'
A voice comes between farts. Then a dance:
Chemo man gathers up his jingling stand
Of tubes and chemicals, embraces it, jigs with it,
'Do you come here often?' Unplug, plug in,
Unplug, plug in, bed to toilet and back,
Hoping to be safe again with unblocked drip.
Afternoon: chemo man hunched on bed
Vomiting into his cardboard bowl, and I mean vomiting,
Retching and retching until he feel his exhaustion
His very insides coming out. Well
That's normal. Rest, get some sleep.

. . .

GORGO: but who knows? Medieval spheres
Gliding on crystal gimbals could not last
The rough inimical perilous world is better
We rule; you rule; back and forward it goes.
Your hosts, your victims, have their obituaries
Closed in the figure of a hard fought fight.
I leave you with the thought that we too,
We wicked ones, we errant cells
Have held our battle ground for millions of years
Uncounted millions of years.
BEAU: the past is not the future. We are ready
To give you the hardest of hard times.

269

My host is walking gently in the sun.
Will you grit your teeth, and think of her?
We shall surely speak again. Arrivederci.[13]

This poem exposes the difference between the normal cell and the unruly cancer cell. The normal one is just so boring and predictable. Gorgo is different, he stimulates the brain. The description of the ward is powerful, as is the effect of chemotherapy on the patient. The comment on pain by Gorgo – *I have never felt it though I have watched our human hosts give signs – a gasp, a groan, a spasm, a scream* is fascinating. Then Beau describes suffering and what it means to have toxic treatment. This a powerful and emotional poem, based on real experience which can be readily related to by patients and relatives, and the clinical staff.

'Ex-Parte statement on the Project of Cancer', in *Stony Limits and Other Poems* (1934)

This remarkable poem by Hugh MacDiarmid illustrates the complexity of cancer and its management. The following extracts give a glimpse into MacDiarmid's thinking:

YOU say cancer's increasin'
– No juist in me –
And wonder what the reason
For that can be,
Aiblins I can tell you
If you listen a wee.

If I canna juist claim to speak
'Frae the inside' yet
I ken something o' the matter frae 'the growin' end'
   And keep learnin' bit by bit.

. . .

But science has advanced a lot lately
   As a'body kens-or thinks he kens

270

And, put bluntly, to my mind it's nae
    Mere coincidence.

. . .

Ye see what I'm driving at. My inside knowledge tells
My Cancer comes frae vagrant primary germ-cells
Which, instead o' formin a mair or less complete
Embryo or embryoma juist delete
That customary gesture to normal life skip it, and give rise
(Cancer, by crikey, kens nae compromise!)
To a larva or phorozoon o' indefinite
Unrestricted powers of growth. You get
My meaning noo?

. . .

And if I translated the sense o' cancer directly
Into words – O they exist, in Scots – they would be
To almost a'body else like those Berlioz invented
For his Chorus o' Shades and syne repented;
But drunk wi' implacable will and mordacity.[14]

(The reference to Berlioz relates to pure gibberish he wrote for the *Chorus of Shades*).

Patients do have the knowledge and the ability to understand, and it is the responsibility of the clinician (of whatever professional group) to encourage that involvement.

As a further example of the importance of the patient view is that of Jean, a seventy-nine year old central character in James Robertson's book *And the Land Lay Still,* who sets out her feelings on her illness; she is obviously unwell. She is asked by Mike, whose father was Jean's lover many years ago, what is wrong and she refuses to answer. 'I've never seen a doctor in my whole life. I don't believe in doctors'. Mike suggest that she might have cancer and she replies:

'Thanks a lot', she says, then, 'Aye, that's what I think too when I look in the mirror'. He asks why she doesn't find out. 'Find out what? That I'm going to die?' and she continues to smoke, which she says helps.

'What's the alternative? My life taken over by doctors who cut me open, fill me with drugs, blast me with radiotherapy, or all three of the above, my hair falls out, I can't manage on my own here at home. I feel like crap and *then* I die. Delaying tactics that's all. Thank you but no.'

The questions here are what would you do in the same position, or if it was your mother or friend? Jean has made up her mind, what would your decision be?[15]

Angela McSeveney (1964–), was brought up in several places across Scotland and graduated in Arts at Edinburgh University. She has written a number of poems and a book, *Coming out with it*. This short poem describes the finding of a breast lump.

The Lump.[16]

Rolling over on a hot June night
I cradled my breast in my arms.
and felt a hard knot of tissue

I was fifteen
My life rose up in my throat
and threatened to stifle me.

It took three attempts to tell my mother
She promised that my appointment would be
with a woman doctor

A nurse called my name
I didn't have cancer

The stitches in my skin reminded me
of a chicken trussed for the oven

I felt ashamed
that the first man to see
me had only been doing his job.

This astutely observed clinical finding reveals the implications for the young woman.

Defining the determinants of health

The second issue to be discussed are the determinants of health which were outlined at the start of the book:

Biological discoveries
Social factors
Lifestyle
Environment
Health services

It sometimes becomes evident that the power of the narrator is greater than that of the learned professor as some of the following extracts show.

Health and the city

There are whole series of novels which depict the life in inner cities, quite differently from the literature of the 19th century. The realism is palpable. They include novels such as *Wax Fruit* (Guy McCrone, 1947), *Dancing in the Streets* (Clifford Hanley, 1958), *The Prime of Miss Jean Brodie* (Muriel Spark, 1961) *Dear Green Place* (Archie Hind, 1996), *Swing, Hammer, Swing* (Jeff Torrington, 1992), *Trainspotting* (Irvine Welsh, 1993) and James Robertson's novel of modern *Scotland And the Land Lay Still* (2010). Other writings such as *A Scots Quair* (Lewis Grassic Gibbon, 1946), *The Para Handy Tales* (Neil Munro, 1951) and the fascinating novels and stories of Robin Jenkins and Alexander McCall Smith describe other aspects of life in Scotland. Many of them tell stories of violence, poverty and dangerous work environments.

The social issues include, of course, the community and groups within the community. In two of John Buchan's books a small, but important group, are key characters in the plot, The Gorbals Diehards, in *Huntingtower* and *The House of the Four Winds*.[17] They are the adventures of Dickson McCunn, a respectable Glasgow Grocer who is joined, unexpectedly by the Gorbals Diehards, a group of urchins. Because of their social status they are unable to join regular boys groups, such as the Scouts, so they set up their own. Dougal is the Chieftan and Buchan describes him in *Huntingtower*,

> It was a stunted boy, who from his face might have been fifteen years old, but had the stature of a child of twelve. He had a thatch of fiery red hair above a pale freckled countenance. His nose was snub, his eyes a sulky grey-green, and his wide mouth disclosed large and damaged teeth . . . his legs and feet were bare, blue and scratched and very dirty . . .

This is a picture of deprivation and poverty, yet part of a group with spirit and discipline. Three decades after this was written the Gorbals area was the subject of some pioneering work in the community by Geoff Shaw,[18] a Church of Scotland minister, who with others including Richard Holloway,[19] later Bishop of Edinburgh, lived in the community to provide help and support. This was reminiscent of another such venture, the Iona Community, begun in the Govan area of the city in 1938 by the Reverend George MacLeod, (later Lord MacLeod of Fuinary) to assist the unemployed and bring hope to them. It continues to this day.

A considerable list of detective stories set in Scotland illustrate, par excellence, the social environment and the dark side of life come from such authors as William McIlvaney (*Laidlaw*), Glenn Chandler (*Taggart*), and Ian Rankin (*Rebus*).

One of these novels is *No mean City*, by A. McArthur and H. Kingsley Long.[20] It is a novel of razor gangs, violent dance halls, and cramped living conditions, set in Glasgow in the 1920s. Here are two short extracts:

> Then as though driven by the wind, the crowd stampeded left and right at the far end of the hall to leave a clear way for Gus MacLean, shouting curses and brandishing a razor in either hand. One man, unarmed, stands little chance against a razor fighter, but Johnnie Stark was fighting mad and bayonets would not have given him pause. He ran three or four steps and then leaped clear off the floor at big Gus. They fell together with a crash that shook the floor, but Johnnie was on top. Quick as a cat, he regained his

feet and kicked, and kicked again with iron-shod boot, against a defenceless head. Gus lay quite still.

Every bottle brought into that hall was smashed during the fight, which ended only with the arrival of the police-three or four of them swinging drawn batons. Dancers, fighters, men and women, everybody able to run, made a wild rush for the exits, and most of them including Johnnie and Mary, got away.

Later his achievements are publicly recognised.

'Who is this, eh?' exclaimed a young gangster in awed admiration. 'Look at him boys! The Razor King!'

As he finds a home for himself and his partner the Razor King's flat is described:

The front door faced the stairs on the third floor landing. Left and right of the 'single end' were the usual two roomed houses. The one room of Razor King's new home was tolerably 'large' by comparison with the kitchen and living room of his own home. Of course, it had no lavatory and there was no bathroom in the whole of the long, grey, four-storied tenement, or for that matter, in the whole of Crown Street. And yet Johnnie and Lizzie agreed that the 'single end' was a 'pure treat'. The rent was exceptionally low; only five and three pence a week.

A number of modern Scottish novels describe the scene at the present. The most powerful of these is *Trainspotting* by Irvine Welsh.[21] This is a remarkable book, amusing, witty, powerful, reactionary, yet true. Two extracts give a contemporary flavour to the people of Scotland and health:

Lenny went down to the pub and sat at the bar with his Daily Record and a pint of lager. He considered lighting a cigarette, then decided against it. It was 11.04 and he'd had twelve fags already. It was always the same when he was forced to rise in the morning. He smoked far too many fags. He could cut down by staying in bed, so he generally didn't get up until 2 p.m. These

Government cunts were determined, he thought, to wreck both his health and finances by forcing him up so early.

o 0 o

Venters had got HIV infection, like most people in Edinburgh, through the sharing of needles while taking heroin. Ironically, prior to being diagnosed HIV positive, he had kicked the junk, but was now a hopeless pisshead. The way he drank indiscriminately, occasionally stuffing a pub roll or toastie into his face during a marathon drinking bout, meant that his weakened frame was easy prey to all sorts of potentially killer infections. During his period of socialising with me, I confidently prophesied that he would last no time.

Another issue which has ethical, social, lifestyle and medical components is that of pregnancy. In particular, teenage pregnancy has been a feature of health-related concerns for centuries. In a recent novel *Tell Me Where You Are,*[22] Moira Forsyth tells the story of a family with complex relationships, which raises two different ways of dealing with the conseqences of an unwanted pregancy. The first is in a thirty-seven year old unmarried professional woman living in Edinburgh who unexpectantly becomes pregnant. It was a mistake, but she has no hesitiation as to what to do: she will have a termination. The second is in a fourteen year old girl, the first woman's niece, who becomes part of the family. By the time she is fifteen she is pregnant, again a mistake. She, after some doubts, agrees to continue the pregnancy and has a safe delivery. The ethical issues in both are similar, and as the older woman watches the younger woman grow and give birth she regularly questions her own decision. A second Aunt, with whom the girl is living, and who has two teenage boys of her own, is there at the birth, which brings back memories for her. She had a miscarriage many years ago, but the pain returns. The ethical issues are clearly set out and both sides of the debate are presented, as are the social circumstances in which two women become pregnant, and another remembers. Three approaches, termination, acceptance and memories.

Environmental issues

One of the most significant determinants of health is the environment. The quality of air, water and soil are all relevant and some of them have already been raised in the 19th century section.

Hugh MacDiarmid wrote powerfully about the issue of geology and climate change in his poem 'The Bonnie Broukit Bairn' (*Neglected*) written 'For Peggy':

> Mars is braw in crammasy, [crimson]
> Venus in a green silk goun,
> The auld mune shak's her gowden feathers,
> Their starry talk's a when o' blethers,
> Nane for thee a thochtie sparin'
> Earth , thou bonnie broukit bairn!
> -But greet, an' in your tears ye'll drown
> The hail clanjamfrie! [collection][23]

And in his poem, 'On a raised beach' he raises a broader issue:

> What happens to us
> Is irrelevant to the world's geology
> But what happens to the world's geology
> Is not irrelevant to us.
> We must reconcile ourselves to the stones
> Not the stone to us.'[24]

We neglect the earth at our peril, and the language of MacDiarmid powerfully exposes the issues.

The problem with teeth

Scotland has always had a bad record for tooth decay. One of the reasons, eating too many sweet things, is well illustrated in the stories of *Wee Mac-Greegor* by J. J. Bell and first published in 1933.[25] He is a little tearaway, who, whenever there is a problem he needs his 'Taiblet'. This is a reference to a block, or tablet, of a very sweet mixture made from evaporated milk, sugar, butter and whole milk. After the taiblet comes the 'Ile' to help, Ile standing for castor oil, which is used to control all known illnesses. He spends his pocket money on sweets and his favourites are the joob-joobs, ('I canna sleep, I want a joob-joob', is a common request) and barley sugar, mixed with sugar-ally water. He is once given an apple for a present and a penny with which he intends to buy 'broken mixtures' of sweets. Such a mixture of sugary temptations is perfect for ruining teeth!

The importance of role models in health

Much of our health behaviour relates to role modelling, those we admire, associate with, and want to be like. What they eat, smoke and drink. This poem by Liz Lochhead, the current Scottish Makar, comprehensively sums up the situation.

Your Aunties.

Your Auntie was
Famous for being an air hostess
Famous for being a nurse
Famous for being a bloody good sport
Famous for being a Pain in the Erse

. . .

Famous for her perra stoatin pins
Famous for the big blue eyes
Famous for her brass neck
Famous for her mince pies

. . .

Famous for her bra
Famous for her scarlet lipstick
Famous for her scarlet fever
Famous for getting up at weddings and
Singing the Twelfth of Never

. . .

Famous for being a nippy sweetie

Famous for the specs you couldn't get on the NHS

Famous for her driving

Famous for her drinking

Famous for driving your Uncle Freddie to drink

. . .

Famous for her peerie heels

Famous for her fake tan

Famous for her wee man

. . . and

A very well-known phrase or saying

Meaning you are

Welcome to whatever you want is;

Eat up, you're at your Auntie's.[26]

Outlining the role and competence of the doctor

The third issue is to describe more fully the role and competencies of the doctor. It is interesting to note how that role has changed with increasing effectiveness of treatment and at the same time, the increasing sophistication and knowledge of the patient. It is very likely that that role will continue to change and develop, in ways yet to be envisaged. It questions the role of the doctor. Is the doctor a healer, a technician, a friend and comforter, or just someone you call on if you think there is a problem? The answer to the question is of course very relevant in terms of the educational programmes provided for doctors and the other caring professions. The topic of specialisation is especially relevant here.

In *The Citadel* (1937) by A.J. Cronin the central character is Andrew Manson, a St Andrews graduate who works in the Welsh Valleys as a GP then moves to London by the lure of private practice. It has been suggested recently that *The Citadel* might have contributed to the initiation of the NHS in the UK.[27] The novel was first published in 1937 and Cronin's connection with the Welsh Valleys where Aneurin Bevan, an architect of the NHS, was an MP may have been relevant as Cronin also practised there. The book covers quality of practice, inequalities in health and the delivery of services, together with a series of ethical issues. It was widely read and highly influential with the public. The film of the book in 1939 was the most successful film in Britain in that year. It could well have had an influential role.

Earlier in this book (p198) it was noted that in 1855 Dr John Snow recognised a problem of cholera in Soho and took the dramatic step of removing the handle of the Broad Street pump to deal with it; an important public health action. Cronin in the Citadel describes a different but just as effective method of dealing with enteric infections in the mining community in Wales. The problem is the sewer which leaks and causes outbreaks of infection. The doctors have written letters but know that any response will be slow. So they take matters into their own hands and decide to blow up the sewer. They find the explosive from the mines and one night blow it up, and the following week construction of a new sewer began. Mission accomplished.

To return to the story, and an a more trivial note, Dr Manson, the main character, does well in private practice, at least initially, but gets advice from a female patient. She questions him:

'Will you take the advice of a woman old enough to be your mother? Go to a good tailor. Go to Captain Sutton's in the Strand . . . you've told me how much you wish to succeed. You never will in that suit.'[28]

This is an interesting link back to Fergusson's '*Gude braid claith.*'

In *Adventures with a Black Bag* (1943) another of A.J. Cronin's books, Dr Finlay encounters a patent who asks a difficult question of the doctor:

'I want you to tell me how long I have to live'. His face was a study. It might even have amused her, for she smiled faintly before going on. 'I've got consumption – sorry I suppose you'd prefer to say tuberculosis. I'd like you to listen to my lungs and tell me just how long I've got to put up with it'. He could have cursed himself for his stupidity; he had been blind not to see it. Everything was there – the hectic flush, emaciation, the quickened breathing – everything. . . . He rose ... took his stethoscope, and spent a long time examining her chest, though there was little need for lengthy auscultation, the lesions were so gross. 'Go on,' she encouraged him. 'Don't be afraid to tell me.' At last with great confusion, he said. 'You've got perhaps six months.' 'You're being kind' she said studying his face. 'You really mean six weeks.' He did not answer. A great wave of pity swept over him.[29]

In the same stories there is a brief mention of chloroform. A patient presents with a huge swelling of his arm and a major infection in the soft tissues. He is a person with whom he has had some disagreements on other matters. He decides to operate and asks the patient if he can give 'a whiff of chloroform'. 'Not on your life 'says the patient, 'There's no chloroform for me. If you're going to butcher me at a', ye can butcher me without it.' 'But the pain!' says Finlay. To which the patient replies 'Aw! What the hell'. . .Ye know fine well ye're wanting to hurt me, go ahead and see if you can make me squeal. Now's the chance to get a little of your own back.'

Finally from *Adventures of a Black Bag* Finlay is depressed over a young lady friend, and he throws himself into his work, he begins to read the literature again, and finds that things are changing in clinical practice. Because of this reading he is able to identify a newly recognised illness. He has been reading about 'appendicitis' which is the talk of London, Paris and Vienna. He subsequently makes the diagnosis in a young boy and in spite of some doubts he thinks he is right. A young colleague has to be consulted to confirm the diagnosis, but he does not agree. The boy continues to deteriorate. 'Here in this poor squalid home, he felt himself faced with the angel of death, he must do something.' He rings up a professor in Glasgow, who has just left on a train for the south of England. He, of course, has to do it himself in the cottage hospital. As expected he finds a gangrenous appendix and removes it, and the patient is saved.

This has been a difficult decision, with significant uncertainty and risk. It also underlines again the value a national health service, and the ability to get effective treatment even if the senior surgeon is on holiday.

In Ian Banks' book *The Crow Road*[30]There is an amusing incident about the doctor. The group are attending a cremation when Dr Fyfe exclaims,

'Ah!' said Dr Fyfe, stumbling just before he was intercepted before the door of the chapel by a concerned undertaker. 'Ah!' he said again, and crumpled, first into the undertaker's arms and then to the ground. He was on his knees briefly, then turned and sat down, clutched at his chest, stared at the granite flagstones outside the chapel, and to the assembled, still stunned and quieted crowd of us announced, 'I'm sorry, folks, but I believe I'm having a coronary . . .' and keeled over on his back.

There was an instant when nothing much seemed to happen. Then Dean Watt nudged me with his hand holding his Regal and said quietly 'There's a funny thing, eh?'

'Dean!' hissed Ashley, as people crowed round the doctor.

'Oo-ya!'

'Call an ambulance!' somebody shouted.

'Use the hearse!' yelled my dad.

'Och, its only a bruise' Dean muttered, rubbing vigorously at his shin. 'Ooya! Will ye *quit* that!'

They used the hearse, and got Doctor Fyfe to the local hospital in ample time to save his life if not his professional reputation.

The muffled crump – which I maintain that I heard – was my grandmother exploding. Doctor Fyfe had neglected to ask the hospital to remove her pacemaker before she was cremated.

Communication skills

The textbooks used by students and doctors also illustrate the changes which have occurred in education and learning. The extract that follows comes from a manual of clinical skills, widely used in the 1960s.

Interrogation of the patient

The medical student uses numerous texbooks and workbooks to assist in learning. One of these used in the late 1950s was Hutchison's *Clinical Methods* (1960 reprint). This comes from the first chapter on 'Case-Taking':

The object of interrogation is to elicit information regarding the patient's present illness, the state of his previous health and that of his family. The interrogation must be patiently carried out, the patient being allowed, as far as possible, to tell his story in his own words. One patient is a good witness and another poor. One gives an excellent history. Another has to have the history of his illness dragged out of him by methods of slow extortion and even then a great of what he says may prove irrelevant. Some patients seem quite unable to give a precise account of what they feel to be wrong. This may be due to stupidity or to the effects of disease on their mental faculties.[31]

This is not necessarily the best approach to adopt in communicating with patients.

Telling the truth is always difficult when the clinical condition is complex and the outcome uncertain. In *Harry Potter and The Philosophers Stone* (1997) by J K Rowling, Dumbledore, the Headmaster, speaks to Harry Potter, the main character:

> 'The truth,' Dumbledore sighed, 'It is a beautiful and a terrible thing, and should therefore be treated with great caution. However, I shall answer your questions unless I have a good reason not to, in which case I beg you to forgive me, I shall not of course lie.'[32]

Telling the truth

John Buchan's book *Sick Heart River*[33] tells the story of Sir Edward Leithen, a distinguished lawyer, who at the beginning of the book is settling his affairs. He is clearly unwell with a chest complaint, he is lethargic and conscious of the frailty of his own body. He goes to his own lawyer to sort out his will, and his legal clerk to finalise his last few cases. He then, in trepidation goes to see Dr Croke, his physician, to demand a final verdict

> The great doctor gave it: gravely, anxiously, tenderly, as to an old friend but without equivocation. He was dying, slowly dying.
>
> Lethan's mind refused to bite on the details of his own case with its usual professional precision. He simply accepted the judgement of the expert. He was suffering from advanced tuberculosis, a retarded consequence of gas poisoning . . .
>
> 'How long have I to live?' he asked, and was told a year, perhaps a little longer.

'Shall I go off suddenly, or what?' The answer was that there would be a progressive loss of strength until the heart failed.

'Can you give me no hope?'

Croke shook his head.

'I dare not. The lesions *might* heal, the fibrous patch *might* disappear, but it would be a miracle according to present knowledge. I must add, of course, that our present knowledge may not be the final truth.'

'But I must take it as such, I agree. Miracles don't happen.'

This is a fascinating conversation, and at the heart of telling the truth to patients and families. Sir Edward leaves Harley Street almost cheerfully, and goes on, in the book, to have a marvellous adventure,

Maintaining competence

Tom Gibson was a distinguished plastic surgeon, past President of the Royal College of Physicians and Surgeons of Glasgow, and a poet. He wrote many poems including, 'Stratified Squamous Skin' and 'Our Undergraduate Medical career'.[34] One of these poems fits well into the continuing learning theme of maintaining competence:

'And Aye there's more to Learn'

'He'd like to be a doctor so
He's soon matriculated
And seven weary years he spends
Ere he's certificated.
There's far too much to learn

He thinks he'd like to specialise
And lord it round the wards
To emulate the giants
Their merited awards
And aye there's more to learn

284

Learning from literature

You've got to get a member- or
A fellow-ship my lad
Or out you go to limbo quick
But please don't look so sad!
We'll show you how to learn

There's basic science lecture and
There's meetings by the score
Courses and symposia
And dear God knows what more
Stick to it lad you'll learn

At last the dreaded days are past
Exams are o'er and done
You fell you've finished training now?
My lad you've just begun!
For aye there's more to learn

By forty-five (if you've behaved)
You're fitted for sole charge,
Deserving utter confidence from
The populace at large
But aye there's more to learn.

You find the modern new ideas
Just slip beyond your reach?
Now's the time to start again
And study how to teach!
So many have to learn

Learning ever learning is
Each good doctor's fate
For knowledge is increasing at
An exponential rate
And aye there's more to learn.[35]

Capturing the patient perspective

A further development from these readings would be to use the texts and examples to give a patient perspective to the discussion; to allow the reader (old or young) to compare and contrast their own views and approach to clinical practice and competence; their own communication skills and ethical approach with that of patients and families, based on what patients say. It also allows questioning of their own wish to be a doctor and to consider how their own role is evolving. Some examples in relation to death and dying may be relevant here.

Death and Dying

These are subjects covered by many authors and allude to both children and adults. James Hogg (1770–1835) wrote a very poignant 'Elegy on the Death of a Child'. Here are the final two stanzas:

> But now I see thee stretched at rest
> To break that rest shall wake no morrow
> Pale as the grave-flower on thy breast
> Poor child of love, of shame, and sorrow.

> My thy long sleep be sound and sweet
> Thy visions fraught with bliss to be
> And long the daisy, emblem meet
> Shall shed its earliest tear o'er thee.[36]

Childbearing and the problems of children loom large in many of the books. For example in *Sunset Song* the birth of Jean Guthrie's daughter is well described.[37] Helen Cruikshank (1886–1975) writes a beautiful prayer for women who cannot bear children:

> Oh, Thou who dost forbear
> To grant me motherhood,
> Grant that my brow may wear

286

Beneath its maiden's snood
Love to distressed Mankind,
And helpful sympathy
For all whom Fate doth bind
In Sorrow's company.

Help me always to choose,
To comfort and to bless,
And in Man's service lose
My fruitful barrenness;
So that my children may
Succour and pity give
To sadder hearts. I pray
O help me so to live.[38]

Hugh MacDiarmid in his poem 'The Glen of Silence' describes the problem of intrauterine death:

Every doctor knows it – the stillness of foetal death,
The indescribable silence over the abdomen then!
A silence literally 'heard' because of the way
It stands out in the auscultation of the abdomen.[39]

His couplet on childbearing and its consequences bears repeating several times. (*A Drunk Man Look at the Thistle,* 1926) 'Millions o' wimnen bring forth in Pain / Millions o' bairns that are no worth ha'en'.[40] And from the same poem, the quest of every doctor; 'I wish I kent the physical basis / O' a' life's seemin' airs and graces.'

The settings of illness are also the subject of a number of important poems and writings, notably by Douglas Dunn (b 1942) in his book *Elegies* (1985, published in memory of his wife).[41] In particular 'Thirteen Steps and the Thirteenth of March' sets the tone:

She sat up on her pillows, receiving guests.
I brought them tea or sherry like a butler,

Up and down the thirteen steps from my pantry.
I was running out of vases.

More than one visitor came down, and said,
'Her room's so cheerful. She isn't afraid'.
Even the cyclamen and lilies were listening,
Their trusty tributes holding off the real.

Doorbells, shopping, laundry, post and callers,
And twenty-six steps up the stairs
From door to bed, two times thirteen's
Unlucky numeral in my high house.

And visitors, three, four, five times a day;
My wept exhaustions over plates and cups
Drained my self-pity in these days of grief
Before the grief. Flowers, and no vases left.

Some sat downstairs with a hankie
Nursing a little cry before going up to her.
They came back with their fears of dying amended.
'Her room's so cheerful. She isn't afraid.'[42]

In Robert McLellan's poem, 'Sweet Largie Bay' (1977) there is a verse
which tells of the mother's concern while the children have a fever:

Through nou to whaur they frettit in their fevers
Here I hae sat through lang lamplicht nichts
Keepin watch ower them in their mumps and measles
My hope hingin hushed on ilka hairt-beat
And wi the fire deein my fear growin[43]

William Soutar was born in 1898 and became a poet having read the work
of Hugh MacDiarmid. He developed ankylosing spondylitis and tuberculosis
and died in 1934, having been bed ridden for four years. He wrote a journal

during this time which was published after his death as *Diary of a dying man*.[44] It is an acutely observed view of impending death. This short poem, from the book, is concerned with diagnosis. D.B. Low, the medico, was William Soutar's doctor. They were friends and had been schoolboys together at Perth Academy, and students together at Edinburgh University. Here he discusses the consultation with the doctor, and the impact on his creativity:

Prospect

'D.B.Low my medico
Pronounced with bedside gravity:
I fear, I fear, that I can hear
The echo of a cavity

Ten days or so, and D.B.Low
With specialist suavity
Soon searches out, beyond a doubt,
The echo of a cavity.

Ten days or so, and so, and so
I find my thoughts' depravity
Begin to hint there is small stint
Of treasure in this cavity.)

It would seem to prove how empty I had become of creative vigour when I could cease from versifying without any regret. It was also a suitable moment with regard to the quantity of verse which I had written during the past three years; the quality was beginning to deteriorate as the making tended to become more mechanical.'

The diaries reflect the patient's changing moods and experiences. For example he records on the 12th May 1942,

Historic day-definitely stopped smoking-not a moral victory, merely the result of the gradual lessening of the pleasure I have had from puffing a cigarette; at last the pleasure has become nil.

> Fare-thee-well
> For many years Tobac and I
> Have been to each a faithful friend;
> And now without a single sigh,
> Our comradeship is at an end.'

Such diaries and related poems and stories, as in *Elegies* by Douglas Dunn quoted above, open up new thinking about the feelings of patients and their families, and provide the clinical professions with learning opportunities.

Patient experiences

Janice Galloway in her book *The Trick is to Keep Breathing* (1989) provides a fascinating account of anorexia and the problems associated with illness.[45] Of particular interest is the way she is looked after by the clinical staff. Here is how she describes an appointment:

Seven minutes early.

The appointment line snakes out the door and into the drizzle. I go to Dr Stead too often and feel bad about it. I always think I am wasting his time and I hate that visits are acrimonious. So I always go early and make notes. It is supposed to make me seem business like and brisk. It is supposed to save his time and my anxiety about it, but it never works out like that. It works out like this:

Doctor: How are things/what's new/ how's the week been treating you?

I try to remember the things in the notepad. They get jumbled and I think I'm going to cry. This is terrible so I don't say anything.

Patient: I'm not sleeping. I'm still not sleeping.

Doctor: Try taking the tallow things an hour earlier in the evening. And the red things later. There's nothing left to do on the green things on this theme. Keep them as they were. [Already writing prescription] Do you need more?

Patient: Thank you. I feel terrible.

Doctor: Well, let's leave it for a while, see how you are next week. One thing at a time, eh?

I come out like a steamrollered cartoon: two-dimensions to start with then flattened some more until I am tissue. I walk to the bus stop with my head down. Even on warm days I take a scarf to hide my face.'

She has been admitted to hospital and the second consultation is even more interesting.

'The doctor is over an hour late. An entirely different man to Dr Two. But questions involve risk and I don't want to look picky. I follow him down the sea-coloured corridor to a room with no pictures and all the curtains closed. It smells like dog in the rain. Dr Three does not waste any time.

Dr Three: [sitting] Well?

Leather elbow patches on his horrible jacket glint in the gloom. Behind the specs his eyes are all gloom.

Patient: [Mesmerised] Well what? I thought you would start?

Doctor Three: Start what? Start What? You asked to see me. You are the one who knows what this is about.

Patient: I've been here nearly a week

Dr Three: Yes. So what can I do for you?

Patient [Confused. Has he forgotten or trying to remember] Treatment. I want to know about treatment.

Dr Three: [Leans back with an Ominous creak] I don't know what sort of thing you expected. There's no set procedure for these things. You ask to see one of us when you feel you need to. So. Any other questions?

Patient: I have to think [Silence]

Dr Three: Well?

Patient: [Nothing, Eyes filling up]

Dr Three: [Draw a long breath through nose, leaning back on chair] How long have you been here did you say?

Patient: Nearly a week, I haven't seen any one.

Dr Three: [Sighing] I suppose you want a pass. [Silence] To go home for the weekend? You should be going home on a pass. Getting out of here and facing up to things on the outside. You can go out on a pass any time you like, all right?

Patient: I don't understand any of this.

Dr Three: I don't know what that's supposed to mean

Patient: It's too fast. You're rushing me.

Dr Three: All right. Take your time. [Silence] Right then good day.

He lifts the bundle of papers on his desk, then folds his arms. The interview is finished.
PATIENT stands thinking maybe this is some kind of therapy.

Dr Three: The interview is over [opens a drawer. The stack of papers flake dangerously. He pretends not to notice.]

Then a final comment by the patient a little later:

'I should refuse to see Dr Three again. He always makes things worse. My notebook will be better than a doctor. I have to learn to minister to myself and let the slogans teach me something. May be that was the idea all along.'

It is difficult not to read such extracts without thinking about how the consultation could have been improved. There is little in the way of empathy, or of skills in communication – indeed Dr Three seems actually hostile to the patient! The doctors misinterpret, and expect the patient to have the answers. The different doctors have different styles, each representing quite different approaches. The conversation acts as a trigger point for further debate and discussion.

How professionals learn

The final issue, especially for policy makers, has already been alluded to, that of preparing people to enter the clinical professions. If you were designing a curriculum or a course for the doctor of the future, what would it look like? What would the knowledge base be and how much time, if any, would be devoted to the humanities? This is a significant issue at the start of the 21st century. We know that the knowledge base will grow exponentially and that teaching of the factual knowledge provided at medical school may be out of date in a few years. This is in complete contrast to, for example, the 18thcentury where the knowledge grew only slowly. We also know that patients and the public will know more and expect more, and that the clinician–patient relationship might change.

It is also equally obvious that social and environmental determinants of health will continue to pose problems, and may become even more relevant. Who should take the lead, in tackling such new and potent risks? Perhaps a consideration of the writings of novelists and poets might add to that debate.

Creative writing

Over the past decade a number of initiatives have been developed to consider the potential of creative writing for both patients and professionals. These include workshops in medical education,[46] its use in palliative care,[47] in exploring clinical practice,[48] and in public health.[49] A number of courses are available for a wide range of staff to examine their own attitudes and feelings about particular issues. The role of the diary, to be reviewed on a regular basis, allows reflection of events and individual clinical issues. Such reflective learning is increasingly common. For patients, similar initiatives can once again allow feelings and emotions to surface and be considered appropriately.

The commonplace book

We return again to the use of the commonplace book in improving our understanding of health and the care given to patients. Such a collection of writings can also be of relevance to patients and the public in helping to make decisions about their lives and their health.

Conclusions

The extracts provided above have been chosen to stimulate discussion and debate with professional staff. In practice, particularly in a small group setting, almost any of the pieces chosen spark argument and provide an opportunity for the individual to consider again their own views and to contrast these with others. Inevitably there will be differences of view, and one of the lessons to be learned is that such differences occur in the real world, in clinical practice. Students and more senior staff need to become aware of this and to recognise that they might have to deal with a decision, or a consultation process with which they may profoundly disagree. They may find themselves in opposition to their senior colleagues, and the need to think through, analyse the problem and be able to articulate their own views clearly and concisely.

This then is the opportunity, to discuss such issues in a supportive environment, and work though their own views on complex clinical and ethical problems. The use of literature can provide one such a route for professional staff.

Notes

1   Calman, *Storytelling, Humour and Learning*.

2   Neil M. Gunn, *The Silver Darlings* (London: Faber and Faber, 1978).

3   J.R. Paterson, 'Castle of Healing', in *Random Rhymes* (Clydebank: Clydebank Press, 1948), p. 40.

4   Eric Linklater, *White-Maa's Saga* (London: Jonathan Cape, 1937).

5   Alasdair Gray, *Poor Things: Episodes from the Early Life of Archibald McCandless M.D., Scottish Public Health Officer* (London: Bloomsbury, 2002).

6   Ian Banks *The Wasp Factory* (London: Macmillan, 1984).

7   Jimmy Black, 'Real Life from Yellow Wednesday', in *Real Life from Yellow Wednesday* (Glasgow: Glasgow District Libraries, 1988), p. 42.

8   James Bridie, *The Sleeping Clergyman and Other Plays* (London: Constable and Co., 1950).

9   'Epistle to John Lapraik,' in *The Complete Works of Robert Burns*, pp. 101–4, ll. 55–72.

10 Robin Jenkins, *The Cone-Gatherers* (Edinburgh: Canongate, 2004).

11 Hugh MacDiarmid *Selected Poetry,* eds. Alan Riach and Michael Grieve (Manchester: Carcanet Press,1992), p. 167 and Hugh MacDiarmid, *Second Hymn to Lenin and other poems* (London: Stanley Nott,1935).

12 Adam McNaughton, 'Cholesterol', http://mysongbook.de/msb/songs/c/choleste. html (04/12/2013).

13 Edwin Morgan, 'Gorgo and Beau', in *A Book of Lives* (Manchester: Carcanet, 2007), pp.56–64.

14 Hugh MacDiarmid, 'Ex-Parte Statement on the Project of Cancer', from *Stony Limits and Other Poems* (1934), in *Complete Poems*, ed. Michael Grieve and W.R. Aitken (Manchester: Carcanet, 1993), pp. 444–9.

15 James Robertson, *And the Land Lay Still*, (London: Penguin Books, 2010), pp. 32–33.

16 Angela McSeveney, 'The Lump' in *Dream State, the New Scottish Poets*, ed. Donny O' Rouke, 2nd ed. (Edinburgh: Edinburgh University Press, 2002), p. 217.

17 John Buchan, *Hunting Tower* (London: Hamlyn Paperbacks, 1982,1st pub. 1922), *The House of the Four Winds*, (Stroud: Alan Suton, 1993 1st pub. 1935)

18 Ron Ferguson, *Geoff*, (Gartocharn: Famedram Publishers, 1979).

19 Richard Holloway, *Leaving Alexandria*, (Edinburgh: Canongate, 2012).

20 A. McArthur and H. Kingsley Long, *No Mean City* (London: Corgi Books, 1957).

21 Irvine Welsh, *Trainspotting* (London: Minerva, 1996).

22 Moira Forsyth, *Tell me where you are.* (Ross-shire: Sandstone Press, 2010).

23 Hugh MacDiarmid, 'The Bonnie Broukit Bairn', from *Sangshaw* (1925), in *The Hugh MacDiarmid Anthology*, eds. Michael Grieve and Alexander Scott (London: Routledge and Kegan Paul, 1975), p. 3.

24   Hugh MacDiarmid, 'On a Raised Beach', from *Stony Limits and Other Poems* (1934), in *The Hugh MacDiarmid Anthology*, pp. 166–7, ll. 212–24.

25   J. J. Bell, *Wee MacGreegor* (Edinburgh and London: The Moray Press, 1945).

26   Liz Lochhead, 'Your Aunties', in *The Colour of Black and White* (Edinburgh: Polygon, 2005), pp. 29–31.

27   S. O'Mahony 'A.J. Cronin and *The Citadel*: did a work of fiction contribute to the foundation of the NHS?', *J.R.Coll. Physicians*, 42 (2012), 172–8.

28   A. J. Cronin, *The Citadel* (London: Hodder and Stoughton, 1961), p. 245.

29   A.J. Cronin, *Adventures of a Black Bag* (London: New English Library, 1979), pp. 20–21.

30   Ian Banks, *The Crow Road* (London: Abacus, 1993).

31   D. Hunter and R.R. Romford, *Hutchison's Clinical Methods*, 13th edn (London: Cassell, 1956), p. 2.

32   J.K. Rowling, *Harry Potter and the Philosopher's Stone* (London: Bloomsbury, 1997), p. 216.

33   John Buchan, *Sick Heart River* (Harmondsworth: Penguin Books, 1985). Originally published posthumously in 1941.

34   Tom Gibson, *Poems and Versifications* (Glasgow: [n.p.], 1991).

35   Tom Gibson, 'And Aye There's More to Learn', in *Poems and Versifications*, pp. 28–32.

36   James Hogg, 'Elegy on the Death of a Child', in *Blackwood's Edinburgh Magazine*, 2.7 (1817), p. 47, ll. 37–44.

37   Lewis Grassic Gibbon, *A Scots Quair: A Trilogy of Novels* (London: Hutchison, 1982), pp. 146–7.

38   Helen Cruickshank, 'A Prayer', in *The Penguin Book of Scottish Verse*, p. 424.

39   Hugh MacDiarmid, 'The Glen of Silence', in *The Hugh MacDiarmid Anthology*, p. 225, ll. 9–12.

40   Hugh MacDiarmid, 'A Drunk Man Looks at the Thistle', in *The Hugh MacDiarmid Anthology*, pp. 23–102, ll. 29–30.

41   Douglas Dunn, *Elegies* (London: Faber and Faber, 1985).

42   Ibid, 'Thirteen Steps and the Thirteenth of March', p. 13.

43   Robert McLellen, 'Sweet Largie Bay', in *Sweet Largie Bay and Arran Burn: Two Poems in Scots* (Preston: Akros Publications, 1977), p. 5–44, ll. 25–29.

44   Soutar, *Diaries*.

45   Janice Galloway, *The Trick is to Keep Breathing* (London: Vintage Books, 1999).

46   S.E. Gull, R.O'Flynn, and J.Y.L.Hunter, 'Creative Writing Workshops for Medical Education', *Medical Humanities*, 28 (2002), 102–4.

47   E. Haraldsottir , 'Poetry and Creative Writing in Palliative care', *British Medical Journal*, Supportive and Palliative Care, 1 (2011), 260.

48   Gillie Bolton, *The Therapeutic Potential of Creative Writing* (London and Philadelphia: Jessica Kingsley Publisher, 1999).

49   Stephen Clift, 'Creative Arts as a Public Health Resource: Moving from Practice-based Research to Evidence-based Practice', *Perspectives in Public Health*, 132 (2012), 120–127.

CHAPTER 17

To see oursels as ithers see us!

The title of this chapter reflects the purpose of the book, that is, to use the literature of Scotland as a way of better understanding the role of medicine, the determinants of health, how they affect us all, and the means of improving both; to get an outside view on health, medicine, quality of life and well-being. Its conclusions are relevant to professionals, patients and the public and the body politic.

It is also relevant to note the lines which follow after the quotation from Robert Burns in the chapter heading,

> *'and wad frae monie a blunder free us*
> *An foolish notion:*[1]

To 'see oursels as ithers see us' may mean changing our behaviour and doing the right thing!

A strong message from the literature of Scotland is that we have known about factors which affect our heath for a very long time. If we just listened and acted, then things might change, for both individuals and the population. There is real potential to improve health

This book has considered a specific part of the literature of the world, Scottish literature, and focussed on a particular aspect, Makars and Mediciners, poets and doctors. In the libraries of the world, big and small, general and specific, there is an enormous resource for teaching, learning and enjoyment. This resource is freely available and can enhance and improve quality of life by providing stimulation and interest for all groups of people. Book clubs and reading groups bring people together, stimulate discussion and build friendships. In professional terms the journal clubs and publication reviews perform a similar function. In the same way the genesis of this book brought staff and students together to learn and enjoy. One of the most striking aspects of such groups, or when speaking about the subject, is the response. Almost without fail at the end of a session, or a seminar, there will be several suggestions as to what to read, or an allusion to another work, usually more relevant than the one used, or an email next day suggesting something else to consider. It is uplifting and enjoyable. For several years after the first student group met I received notes from students suggesting works to read. Inevitably the choice of readings and authors here is restricted and represents my personal preferences. One of the tasks for the reader of this volume is to identify other books, poems and plays which would be both relevant and inspirational.

At the beginning of this book a series of questions were set out which it is appropriate to review and to discuss whether or not they have been answered. This chapter also allows some more general conclusions to be drawn.

The extracts of Scottish literature in the various time periods illustrate the wealth of material available. They suggest that clinical practice has been adequately covered and emphasise how much there is in the literature about health, illness and medicine. The readings have illustrated the very wide range of topics covered including health, quality of life, and in particular attitudes to death and dying.

In addition, the readings show just how contemporary even the older works are in relation to the promotion of health. For example, John Armstrong's poem in the 18th century, 'The Art of Preserving Health', could be a model for a public health programme in the 21st Century. Later, health-related extracts, confirm this. We know what causes bad health, and have known it for centuries, but individuals and communities don't seem to act on the advice and the knowledge available. Of course we need to know more, and recent advances in genetics, for example, which allow sub-sets of the population with particular risks to be identified, have resulted in the possibility of new and more sophisticated methods of prevention to be determined. What is clear, however, is that there is the potential to improve the health of the population now, if individuals were able to take relatively simple steps to change behaviour in relation to diet, exercise, smoking, alcohol and drugs. This is an important conclusion.

This concept was reviewed in 1998 in a short book, *The Potential for Health,* and the basic principle still stands, that there is a huge potential to improve health with existing knowledge.[2] The question asked by Burns in his 'Address to the unco guid, or the rigidly righteous' remains valid and perhaps even more relevant in the 21st century: 'One point must still be strangely dark/ the moving why they do it.' The knowledge to improve health is available, and will undoubtably be augmented with time, so perhaps the real research question is about how we change behaviour using the health knowledge we already have. To quote Burns again: 'But human bodies are such fools/ for a' their Colleges and schools'.[3] It's not just knowledge that matters; people, and populations, have to want to change. It must be seen to be worthwhile for them personally. Putting together the potiential to improve health and the power of the word and the arts generally to change behaviour, I put forward a proposal, some years ago, to consider the arts as a mechanism to improve health.

The contagious theory of behaviour change

The bacillus of laughter is a difficult bug to isolate: once brought under the microscope it will turn out to be a yeast-like ferment equally useful in making wine or vinegar or bread. Arthur Koestler in *The Act of Creation*[4]

In a book written in 2000 I made the case for a contagious agent, the Transmid, being the mechanism by which behaviour could be changed using humour or stories.[5] The story is the agent itself, and I developed the idea of the Transmid – the transmitted idea – being analogous to an infectious agent. The assumption was that people could be changed by stories, and Gardner (1995) in his study of leadership showed how great leaders used stories to change policies, and thinking. The idea that change in learning is 'caught, not taught' is not a new one, nor is the concept of infection in this context. As Shakespeare said in *Anthony and Cleopatra* 'The nature of bad news infects the teller', or Scott in *Harold the Dauntless*, '. . . the romancer's tale becomes the reader's dream.' The *Meme Machine*

300

by Susan Blackmore (1999)[6] suggests that what makes us different is our ability to imitate. Thus the Transmid is used to describe the mechanism by which ideas, behaviour, knowledge and information are transmitted from one person to another, very similar to Osler's 'Mind to Mind'. Interestingly Samuel Cohn recently published a Chapter on 'the Epidemiology of the Black Death and Successive waves of Plague'[7] in which he makes that point that 'Before 1348 the word *contagium* (contagion) was rarely used , especially outside the medical profession. When chroniclers and theologians used the term, it applied almost exclusively to heresy or revolt and not to diease.'

The analogy can be developed further in that some Transmids will be very virulent, and thus very effective in change, others less contagious. The recipients may be sensitive, or resistant, to a particular Transmid. Indeed in some people there may be initial susceptibility but then resistance develops. Bad habits return after a period of abstinence and while the idea may be effective at first this then wears off. In this book many examples have been given of writings (stories) which could change both attitudes and behaviour. Perhaps one of the roles of the storyteller in relation to health is to change people and communities, and perhaps we should have an annual prize for the best story, poem, or work of art which has the potiential to change or behaviour and or health. The power of the word is essential in the shaping of the message. The arts generally are effective, and cartoons, one of my special interests, particularly potent.

Traditionally, of course, the media and advertising are ways to change behaviour, and the newer social media had added to this. Some time ago the World Health Organisation's European office held a symposium entitled 'The pen is as mighty as the Surgeon's scalpel'[8] which set out to look at health messages in the press.

What is striking is just how much things have changed. The patterns of disease seen in the 21st century in Scotland are significantly different from other centuries. Until relatively recently infection was the major cause of death, now it is a range of chronic dieases dominated by heart disease, stroke and cancer. People are living longer: for example, data from the General Register of Scotland (2009) shows that in 1861 the average life span for males was 40.3 years and 43.9 years for females. By 2004–2006 this had risen to 74.6 and 79.6 years respectively. The Scottish Public Health Observatory (2013) records that between 1980 and 2010 life span rose from 75.1 years in women to 80.6 years and in males from 68.7 to 76.3 years. The implications of this basic information are enormous: a larger population with complex illness and an increasingly elderly population. Add to this the new range of treatments and diagnostic investigations available and there is an immediate problem in developing staff and ensuring that they provide a service which is of high quality and which retains the values of care and compassion.

There are thus several aspects which merit further reflection. First, I have focussed attention on the role of the doctor, the skills and competencies required and the way in which the role has changed over the years, from the country doctor in the 16th or 17th century with very little therapy available; to the doctor in the 18th century where new methods were just beginning to be used; to the 19th century doctor, described in the 'Kailyard' literature in glowing terms; to the doctor of today, juggling with a wide range of new treatments and diagnostic aids, but still requiring compassion and a professional approach to ethical issues and communication. The doctor is now described in a more critical and realistic way as, for example, in the Dr Finlay stories or in one of the many television representations of clinical practice. Increasing specialisation is a key feature of modern medicine which makes an holistic approach to looking after the patient more difficult. The importance of discovery and curiosity have been emphasised already in this book. Keeping abreast of new developments is critical and as the good Dr McLure said as he was dying 'a'did what a'cud to keep up to date, but a' hed little time for reading' (p.165). The new doctor will have to do better. A major change in the last century has been the rise in the percentage of women in medicine, now greater than that of men.

The provision of a health service has radically changed over the last few centuries, from none at all, to the modern National Health Service which now provides universal coverage and is free at the point of need. This is one of the striking features of the change over the years. In Scotland, the advent of the National Health Service on the 5th May 1948 changed everything for the population, and it remains a cornerstone of improving health and quality of life. This in itself is an important conclusion. One of the earliest documents cited was *A Satyre of the Three Estates,* in which John the Common-Weal is brought into the political system to change the lot of those who are disadvantaged.

There is also little doubt that the context, social and political, in which the writing on health issues took place, affects the way in which the issues are described. The most obvious one noted here is the paucity of writing in the literature of Scotland, in poems and novels, on poverty and industrialisation in the second half of the 19th century. This is a key point and requires further analysis and confirmation.

A further question at the heart of this debate is whether or not medical values have changed. This is more difficult to assess as very much more is expected of the doctor in the 21st century, and the knowledge base has expanded so much. Patients, quite properly, are much more informed and have greater access to information from a very wide range of sources. While doctors still rank highly in public opinion, the gap between the doctor and the patient has significantly narrowed. New approaches are therefore required if the quality of care is to be maintained. In any professional group the value base needs to be assessed regularly. The evidence presented in this review of the literature of Scotland allows that external perspective to be drawn (*To see oursels as ithers see us*), and through poems and stories encourage reflection on the past, and the present. The values of a profession set out in chapter two remain valid today, and are underscored by this literature review.

A particular aspect of the doctor's role is in the care for patients and families in times of dying and bereavement. In one sense this is a touchstone of the clinical role. In therapeutic terms there has been some progress in this area. There are better analgesics and anxiolytics, and the nursing quality has improved considerably over the centuries, but in nothing quite as radical as in other clinical areas, such as oncology or in the treatment of cardiovascular disease. However, much of the effort in the management of death and dying remains at the personal level, between the patient/family and the clinician. This interaction, at the heart of professionalism, is one which might be followed in more detail to assess the changing quality of care. Improving quality of life for patients, families and communities has been a recurring theme.

It is also relevant to consider how writers have viewed the doctor, and how this has changed. There is little doubt, as some of the extracts in the previous chapter demonstrate the public's views on doctors are not always favourable. Indeed there is a significant shift from the earlier period where the doctor is a key and respected figure in the community, to the 21st century where overt criticism is common. Such examples compel the professional to think again about their own practice and modify this as appropriate. The examples can be used as significant learning experiences.

The second issue relates to quality of life and happiness and how they have been defined over the centuries. This book began with an extract from Barbour's 'The Bruce' in which the evocation of personal freedom is set out, an important component of happiness. Henryson's comment in the 'Tale of the Country mouse and the Town Mouse' is mirrored by Ramsay in 'The Gentle Shepherd', 'He that hath just enough can soundly sleep', or with Fergusson in 'Ode to the Gowdspink', 'While he that gangs wi' ragged coat, is weel contentit wi' his lot.' Burns is even stronger in 'The Epistle to Davie': 'It's no in titles nor in rank/ It's no in wealth like Lon'on Bank/To purchase peace and rest'. Burns also makes the point in 'Tam o' Shanter' that happiness and quality of life don't just come to you, you also have to take action: 'Nae man can tether tide or tide, the hour approaches Tam maun ride.' You also have a responsibility for your own well-being. Quality of life is also an individual matter; your quality of life may be different from mine.

To ensure that quality of life and happiness are part of the ethos of the health service I have suggested on a number of occasions that Departments of Health should be renamed The Department of Health and Happiness.

The third issue concerns the determinants of health. Throughout the readings across the centuries a wide range of issues has been raised: diet, alcohol, exercise, social conditions, housing, living standards, slums, the poorhouse, pollution, poverty and disease, education and employment. Barbour's 'freedom' is also relevant here.

There is a clear political dimension to these determinants, as well as a medical one, hence the importance of the doctor and other health professionals as advocates of change. It was a Glasgow woman weaver who said it most succinctly;

Ask then what is the meaning of the word politics? Is it not the best way to make people happy? 1830, *The Northern Star*

A key purpose of this book was to assess whether a 'commonplace book' might have a role in medical education and in the shaping of the next generation of doctors. Increasingly in medical schools, the arts are seen to have a place, and literature is only one part of this wider spectrum. As medicine becomes more and more technical, science based and evidence driven, there remains a need to assert the humanity of medicine, and the importance of caring and compassion. For many young doctors this will be through the example of their seniors and teachers; role models are critical. But with more and more frequent rotations and changing specialities, and increasing specialisation, it may be more difficult to have an effective mentorship/ apprenticeship process. The use of literature, and this volume emphasises the particular role of Scottish literature, can provide a way of raising difficult issues, allowing discussion and the challenging of assumptions and behaviours. Creative writing adds another dimension to this process. Such issues can be difficult to cover in a busy clinical practice, when there is a need for time to reflect and consider. My own commonplace book has been used, in addition, to collect thoughts and ideas for writing and reflection as noted above.

In some instances such professional issues might best be considered outside a particular clinical speciality, for example as part of the teaching of ethics, where there is space and an environment which encourages such debate. In other instances the bedside might well be the best, with real patients and real problems. However, learning in medicine does not stop at undergraduate level and there is a need to continually review and update skills and competencies. A process of re-validation and regular assessment is now mandatory. While courses and skills-based learning are available, it remains essential that the wider values of being a doctor are promoted. In more modern times the role of science programmes, films, television, and magazines featuring clinical stories and dramas, have served to provide even more in the way of role models and information about the services and their quality which are available. Their realism, accuracy and ethos may, or may not, always be appropriate, but they are widely viewed and read and can change public opinions and behaviour. There is also a place for more multi-disciplinary learning, bringing together the sciences, medicine and the arts. In a phrase used earlier in this book (*Beside the Bonnie Brier Bush*) there is value in a 'commonwealth of letters' (p.164) where a wide variety of different perspectives are presented.

One further feature which emerges is the way in which numerous connections are noted between authors, and between doctors and authors. A number of instances have been identified where such links occur and these have sometimes changed the delivery of the service. The clearest example is that following the tragic death of Robert Fergusson in 1774. His doctor and friend, Andrew Duncan, determined that things would get better and he set out to change public opinion, and raise funds to build the Edinburgh Asylum, which he achieved. Another might be the story, related in an obituary, where Robert Louis Stevenson tells his physician, Thomas Bodley Scott, that he has had an idea for a new adventure story, *Treasure Island*. These connections between authors and doctors also illustrate the breadth of interest of many doctors, outside medicine. This may well assist in giving a different perspective to health and healing.

Some final reflections

Much of this book is about recording the changes and developments of both the clinical professions and the public in relation to health, and how literature might assist in improving the knowledge and understanding for both groups.

A more fundamental question is whether literature has any purpose or role beyond entertainment and enjoyment, in changing health. It has already been suggested above, that literature could have such a role, in alerting the public of dangers to health of particular behaviours. This is not a new role for literature to have a campaigning edge. Consider the response to the question posed in Aristophanes' play *The Frogs* (405 BC). 'Why do we need a poet? To save the city of course.'[9] Thus literature and the arts may also help to improve heath.

It is perhaps here that the role of literature and the arts generally can have an advantage, by the author exposing poor health choices and behaviour patterns, in ways which are more powerful and effective than those of the medical teacher or professor. The writer's imagination and expression can change things. The word can be powerful. The blend of knowledge and creativity can assist in changing behaviour. The examples from the field of cancer given in previous chapters ('Rab and his Friends', in Chapter 13, p177, 'The House with the Green shutters', in Chapter 14, p219, and the two poems on cancer by Edwin Morgan in Chapter 16, p268 and Hugh MacDiarmid in Chapter 16, p270) illustrate just how powerful a personal reflection can be if delivered by someone whose special interest is in the written word. Patients themselves, and patient organisations, are also powerful advocates for change and improvement on the care given.

A second quotation which might add to this discussion comes from Hugh MacDiarmid from his poem 'A Drunk Man Looks at the Thistle' (1926):

> The function, as it seems to me,
> O' poetry is to bring to be
> At lang, lang last that unity . . .[10]

MacDiarmid takes this thought even further in his poem 'Poetry and Science'.[11] He begins the poem with a quotation from Sir Ronald Ross, a Nobel Prize winner (1902) for his work on malaria.

Poetry and Science
Science is the Differential Calculus of the mind,
Art is the Integral Calculus; they may be
Beautiful apart, but are great only when combined.
Sir Ronald Ross

The rarity and value of scientific knowledge
Is little understood – even as people
Who are not botanists find it hard to believe
Special knowledge of the subject can add
Enormously to the aesthetic appreciation of flowers!
Partly because in order to identify a plant
You must study it very much more closely

Than you would otherwise have done, and in the process
Exquisite colours, proportions, and minute shapes spring to light
To small to be ordinarily noted.

Wherefore I seek a poetry of facts

Without some chemistry one is bound to remain
Forever a dumbfounded savage
In the face of vital reactions
Shown only by biochemistry
Replace a stupefied sense of wonder
With something more wonderful
Because natural and understandable.
Nature is more wonderful
When it is at least partly understood
Such an understanding dawns
On the lay reader when he becomes
Acquainted with the biochemistry of the glands
In their relation to disease such as goitre
And their effects on growth, sex and reproduction
He will begin to comprehend a little
The subtlety and beauty of the action
Of enzymes, viruese, and bacteriophages,
These substances which are on the borderland
Between the living and the non-living

The lines 'Nature is more wonderful/When it is at least partly understood'
indicate a profound philosophy of the links between science and the arts,
between poetry and medicine.

It is possible that this could be one of the purposes of the use of literature in health and medical education, to help to bring unity between
the arts and the sciences, allowing new ideas to emerge and to influence
thinking and behaviour; to allow a synthesis of two different ways of
thinking: to encourage the clinician and the artist to work together to
improve understanding. Thus by using the warp and the woof of these two

different approaches to human existence, both might benefit, and the lives of people improved.

Perhaps an old phrase in a different context might help to illuminate this discussion. This would be to develop a new Caledonian antisyzygy (i.e. the ability to see things in different ways), a phrase first used in G. Gregory Smith's book, *Scottish Literature: Character and influence* and develop a *Medical Antisyzygy*.[12] Gregory Smith's concept signified that it was possible to view an idea from two different perspectives; Science, medicine and the arts working co-operatively for the improvement of all – a medical antisyzygy.

And perhaps that is a further main conclusion; the need for a synthesis of the arts, sciences and medicine for the benefit of humanity, a common-wealth of letters.

What can we then conclude from this association between the literature of Scotland and health and medicine? First that it is possible to improve the health of an individual or population using existing knowledge. The values of a profession remain important especially as the knowledge base increases. Second, having a national health service contributes greatly to health and well-being and provides a means by which those who need care can have ready access to services. Quality of life and well-being are at the heart of providing a public service and the examples given throughout this book show how relevant this can be to patients and communities. Third, the context and time in which the writing takes place affect its content, most noteworthy in this study in relation to the lack of works covering poverty and industrialisation in the Victorian era. Fourthly, it recognises that patients and the public have much to contribute to this debate on how to improve health and quality of life.

It also proposes that literature and the arts have a place in the education of the clinical professions. The relevance of the wider interests of doctors, especially in the arts, may give a broader perspective in healing and health. Literature and the arts have a role in improving health. The written and spoken word can be very powerful in changing behaviour.

Finally, there is a case for the unity and integration of the arts and sciences (the warp and the woof) for the benefit of humanity with the development of the concept a medical antisyzygy.

To conclude with a short extract from John Armstrong's poem on 'The Art of Preserving Health'.[13] It encapsulates much of what has been raised in this book. The arts can raise us above grief and pain and as one power, medicine and the arts, come together to improve health and quality of life.

> Music exalts each Joy, allays each Grief
> Expels Diseases, softens every Pain,
> Subdues the rage of Poison, and the Plague;
> And hence the wise of ancient days ador'd
> One Power of Physic, Melody, and Song.

This takes us back to where we began. Effective care for people and their communities requires the fusion, and the power, of science, medicine and the arts. To provide a service based on modern, evidenced-based medicine, the doctor, and the team, will need to provide not only first class diagnostic techniques and therapy, but in addition, access to the arts including dance, drama, music, painting and literature. In this way, care and compassion can be delivered to patients and their families, communities and populations; the person seen as a whole being, *'cut rose-diamond fashion, with many facets.'*[14]

There is still much to read, to learn and to enjoy.

Notes

1 Robert Burns, *To a Louse,* in *The Complete Poetical Works of Robert Burns,* ll. 43–48.

2 Calman, *Potential for Health*

3 Robert Burns. *The Twa Dogs,* in *The Complete Poetical Works of Robert Burns,* ll. 7–8.

4 Arthur Koestler *The Act of Creation*, (London: Hutchison, 1964), p. 32.

5 Calman, *Storytelling, Humour and Learning.*

6 Susan Blackmore, *The Meme Machine,* (Oxford: Oxford University Press, 1999)

7 Samuel Cohn, Medical History Supplement No 27: Pestilential Complexities: Understanding the Medieval Plague, ed Vivian Nutton, (London, 2008) p. 79–80.

8 Symposium, *The pen is as mighty as the Surgeon's Scalpel,* WHO Regional Office, 1988.

9 Aristophanes, *The Frogs* (London: George Allen and Unwin, 1959), p. 101.

10 Hugh MacDiarmid, 'A Drunk Man Looks at the Thistle', *The Hugh MacDiarmid Anthology*, p. 99.

11 Hugh MacDiarmid from *Lucky Poet* (1943) in Selected Poetry by Hugh MacDiarmid, Edited by Alan Riach and Michael Grieve, Caranet Press 1992 p. 196–7.

12 Smith, *Scottish Literature,* p. 4.

13 Armstrong, *Art of Preserving Health,* IV, ll. 514–18.

14 Holmes, *Professor at the Breakfast Table,* p. 29.

APPENDIX 1

Doctors known to Burns

Burns' fame and personality took him into contact with many of the doctors in Scotland at the time. Perhaps his first acquaintance with doctors was while flax-dressing in Irvine where he was known to Dr Hamilton, later referred to as one of the poet's Kilmarnock friends. He subsequently met Dr John MacKenzie when he was twenty-four years of age on his return to Lochea, Tarbolton, during his father's last illness, about the end of 1783.

Dr John MacKenzie of Mauchline

Burns became friends with MacKenzie during his father's illness and the family's removal to Mossgiel. They wrote to each other and dined together, most famously at the dinner table of Professor Dugald Stewart at Catrine. Mackenzie married Helen Miller, one of the Mauchline Belles, and moved to Irvine to practice. He received an MD in Edinburgh for his thesis on 'De Carcinomate' and after moving to Edinburgh died in 1837. It is interesting to note that he presided on the founding of the Irvine Burns Club in 1827, and that Mr David Sillar ('a brother poet') was the vice chair.

Another of the Mauchline Belles, a troup of young ladies referred to by Burns, Miss Smith also married a medical man, Mr James Candlish, whom Burns knew at school in Dalrymple and Ayr. He studied medicine in Glasgow, but was never robust, and moved to Edinburgh as a teacher of medicine. Burns and he corresponded and Burns refers to him as one of his earliest friends though there is no strong evidence that this gave him additional medical knowledge.

The Edinburgh Connection

With the publication of the Kilmarnock Edition, and with the assistance of some friends, Burns was introduced to Edinburgh medical and academic society. It is interesting to note that there were over fifty medical subscribers to the Edinburgh edition, and they are listed as an appendix to this book.[1] Burns met Dr James Gregory, Professor of the Practice of Medicine, and a friendship was begun. Findlay notes that Chambers records their first meeting when Dr Gregory began to ask Burns about his family. ' "Well, Burns" said the physician, "what sort of man was your father – a tall man?" "Yes rather" "and your mother?" "My mother was not a man at all, sir." '[2] Gregory presented him with an English translation of Cicero's select orations, and Burns wrote inside it, 'This book, a present from the truly worthy and learned Dr Gregory, I shall preserve to my latest hour, as a mark of the gratitude, esteem, and veneration I bear the donor. So help me God!'[3] Burns later responded by immortalising him in verse as 'Worthy Gregory's Latin face' in 'Lament for the absence of William Creech, Publisher'.[4]

When Burns was confined to his lodgings for several weeks with an injured knee he was attended by Gregory as his physician and Mr Alexander Wood was the surgeon. This accident took place during the correspondence with 'Clarinda'. Poetry was shared between them, and around the same time the correspondence with Anne Hunter, the wife of John Hunter, became established. John Hunter, born in East Kilbride, had studied medicine in Glasgow and followed his doctor brother William to London where they dominated the London medical scene. Mr Wood (also known as Lang Sandy Wood) had a tall lanky figure. Chambers describes him as 'a man after Burn's own heart-kind, quaint, fond of children and animals.'[5] He even had, like Burns, a pet sheep which trotted after him through Edinburgh. 'Clarinda' (Mrs Agnes McLehose) was also the daughter of a Glasgow surgeon, Andrew Craig, and wrote to Burns about Mr Wood 'I am glad to hear Mr Wood attends you; he is a good soul, and a safe surgeon. I know him a little. Do as he bids, and I trust your leg will soon be quite well.'[6] This is quite a remarkable range of medical men who feature in Burns circles, confirming the social and cultural, as well as the professional importance of doctors in the later 18th century,

Other notable medical names

Of medical men known to Burns one of the most significant was Dr John Moore. He studied medicine in Glasgow and Paris, and practised in Glasgow.

He lived first in Donald's Land, Trongate, opposite the Tron Steeple, and afterwards in Dunlop Street. He was a friend of Tobias Smollett, who was a little older than he was, and who was learning his medical trade in Dr Gordon's surgery in Gibson's land at the corner of Saltmarket and Prince's Street, where Moore had also been an apprentice. Moore travelled to the continent with the 8th Duke of Hamilton, and then settled in London. He wrote a number of works including the novel *Zeluca* (1789), admired by Burns. The pair maintained a correspondence, and Burns wrote eight letters on his side of the exchange. This included his famous autobiographical one dated Mossgeil, 2nd August 1787, which he wrote after his first visit to Edinburgh. The initiation of the correspondence was the letters from Dr Moore to Mrs Dunlop, and she sent Burns extracts of them to see. They shared their interest in literature, and Burns sent him poems to consider. Moore makes the interesting point in one of these letters, 'Why should you by using that (the Scots language) limit the number of your admirers to those who understand Scottish, when you could extend it to all persons of taste who understand the English Language.'[7] Again we see medical men of wide and forceful cultural opinions.

In the middle of this correspondence with Moore, Burns made a visit to Paisley. While in Paisley he met his friend Alex Pattison, a bookseller, when another medical man walked by and recognised Burns from his portrait. This was Dr John Taylor, another doctor with wide acquaintances, and he invited him to his home and they spent an afternoon in conversation. This, in addition, suggests that the portrait of Burns was a good likeness and that he had seen it and read Burns' work.

The letters continued and Moore sent Burns a copy of *Zeluco*. Burns' response to it is interesting and shows a fascinating academic and analytic streak:

> I never take it up without at the same time taking my pencil, and marking with asterisms, parentheses etc., whenever I meet with an original thought, a nervous remark on life and manners, a remarkable, well-turned period, or a character sketched with uncommon precision.[8]

In return for Moore, Burns, in his eighth and last letter enclosed copies of 'Tam o' Shanter', 'Elegy on Captain Matthew Henderson' (1793), and

315

comments on the ballad on the 'Queen Mary'. This letter was dated 28th February 1791 and from Ellisland. They had no further correspondence but Burns continued to hear of him through Mrs Dunlop. Dr Moore was another medical man with a central role in the legend of Burns by widening Burns' reading and commenting on his poems. Another example of the breadth of medical thought at the time.

Burns' doctor in Dumfries, and until the end of his life, was Dr William Maxwell (1760–1834). He was a Jacobite and a Catholic whose father had fought with Prince Charles at Culloden. Maxwell and Burns shared liberal political ideas. Burns paid Maxwell several compliments including the poem to 'Lovely young Jessie' quoted above, and presented the doctor, on his death bed, with a pair of pistols. In addition the poet's youngest child born on the 25th July 1796, the day of his father's funeral, was to be called Maxwell as a mark of respect for the poet's great friend. Maxwell also supplied Dr James Currie with some of the particulars of Burns' illness and death. The method of treatment used by Maxwell on Burns – cold water immersion – has been the subject of much debate and will be discussed later in this chapter.[9]

Another doctor who gave testimony about Burns was Dr John Thomson. At the time of Burns' death in 1796, Thomson was around sixteen years of age and in the same class at Dumfries Academy as the poet's elder son. The pair were said to be on intimate terms and Thomson taught Burns French early on summer mornings. This may have given him insight into Burns' last days. Mr Thomson became tutor to the Gregory family in Edinburgh and then went on to study medicine. There is some evidence that he was present around the time of the death, but as a friend, not the medical attendant.

There was a further wide range of medical contacts in Burns's final years: Dr Mundell practising in Dumfries to whom Burns sent a patient with a complaint in her shoulder; Dr Samuel Hughes of Hereford who was sent a copy of 'Bruce's address to his troops at Bannockburn' (1793); and Dr Robert Watt, later President of the Faculty of Physicians and Surgeons of Glasgow, who lived for a while in Ellisland and had the opportunity to read from Burns' library. This is a fascinating list of medical people associated with Burns and they are a key part of Scottish culture at this period. Across Europe, medicine was pre-eminent in Edinburgh. These practitioners set a long-term example for the profession over the next three centuries and many were part of the Enlightenment.

Dr James Currie

Burns' first biographer, James Currie (1756–1805) was one of the most influential of all Burns' medical contacts. He was born in Kirkpatrick Fleming in Dumfriesshire, and after numerous adventures, including emigrating to Virginia in 1771 studied medicine in Edinburgh, graduating in 1780, and then moved to Liverpool. In 1782 he bought a property in Dumfriesshire and met Burns once, in Dumfries. He was elected a Fellow of the Royal Society, and his main contribution to medicine was a book, which ran to four editions on *Medical reports on the effects of water, Cold and Warm, as a remedy in Fever and Febrile Diseases, whether applied to the Surface of the Body, or used as a Drink, with observations on the Nature of Fever and on the Effects of Opium, alcohol and Inanition* (1805).[10] After Burns' death several people were considered to edit the poet's work and write the biography. Currie's qualifications to do this were minimal and his presentation of Burns as someone with an alcohol problem left an impression that persisted for many years. The four volume edition appeared in 1800, and it went into numerous editions through the rest of the 19th century. There were almost thirty medical subscribers to Currie's first edition.

William Findlay notes:

Without fee or reward, then, and out of pure love for the theme, if the honourable gratification of literary ambition be excluded, this kind hearted physician undertook the task, because nobody else among the poet's many literary friends could be got to do it, 'men of established reputation,' he tells us in his dedication, 'naturally declining an undertaking, to the performance of which it was scarcely to be hoped that general approbation could be obtained, by any exertion of judgement or temper.[11]

Thus this important task was left to a general practitioner based in Liverpool, with little background in literary editing or biography. It required negotiating with Mrs Dunlop, Mrs McLehose and with George Thomson for songs written by Burns, and many others including the family.

Currie's biography has not been without criticism, on two possible grounds, well summarised by Leask.[12] The first relates to his treatment of Burns himself, as someone with problems with alcohol and sexual transgressions, subjects which distressed his admirers. Much of Currie's thinking was based on a theory of health by Dr John Brown (1735–1787) from Edinburgh whose writing and teaching had a major influence on Currie but which were opposite to those of Dr William Cullen (1710–1790), one of the leaders of medicine in Edinburgh. The theory proposed a link between excitement and stimulation, thus to alleviate asthenia, melancholia or depression, stimulation was required using alcohol or opium. The second aspect links Currie's own medical writing, including the paper on 'Medical Reports on the Effects of Water' noted above, to the health of Burns. Currie was also concerned about the management of the poor in Liverpool together with the establishment of a fever hospital and an asylum. He comments on alcohol in terms of the cause of Burns' death, but does not refer to fever or what would now be called rheumatic heart disease. It is this view which has been controversial.

Notes

1   Findlay, *Robert Burns and the Medical Profession*, pp. 32–34 (see Appendix 1, pp. 227–8 of the current book).

2   Ibid, p. 23.

3   Ibid, p. 24.

4   'Lament for the absence of William Creech, Publisher', in *The Complete Poetical Works of Robert Burns*, pp. 277–8, l. 37.

5   Findlay, *Robert Burns and the Medical Profession*, p. 28.

6   Ibid, p. 29.

7   Ibid, p. 45

8   'Letter of Robert Burns to John Moore, 14 July 1790', Griffin, *The Letters of Robert Burns*, p. 45.

9   See Thornton, *William Maxwell to Robert Burns*.

10 James Currie, *Medical reports on the effects of water, Cold and Warm, as a remedy in Fever and Febrile Diseases, whether applied to the Surface of the Body, or used as a Drink, with observations on the Nature of Fever and on the Effects of Opium, alcohol and Inanition*, 4th edn (London: T Cadel and W Davies, 1805).

11   Findlay, *Robert Burns and the Medical Profession*, p. 71.

12   Nigel Leask, 'Robert Burns and the Stimulant Regime' in *Fickle Man: Robert Burns in the 21st century*, eds. J.Rodger and G. Carruthers (Ross-shire: Sandstone Press, 2009), pp. 145–159.

Bibliography

Primary Sources

Alexander, William, *Johnny Gibb of Gushetneuk in the Parish of Pyketillum* (Edinburgh: David Douglas, 1881).

Aristophanes, *The Frogs* (London: George Allen and Unwin, 1959).

Armstrong, John, *The Art of Preserving Health*, 4 vols (London: T Davies, 1774).

Banks, Ian, *The Crow Road* (London: Abacus, 1993).

Barrie, J. M., *Auld Licht Idylls* (London: Hodder and Stoughton, 1934).

—, *The Little Minister* (London: Cassell and Co., 1893).

—, *Peter Pan* (London: Vintage Classics, 2009).

—, *A Window In Thrums* (London: Hodder and Stoughton, 1937).

Beattie, James, *Scoticisms, Arranged in Alphabetical Order Designed to Correct Improprieties of Speech and Writing* (Edinburgh: William Creech, 1797).

Bell, J. J., *Wee MacGreegor* (Edinburgh and London: The Moray Press, 1945).

Black, Jimmy, *Real Life, from Yellow Wednesday* (Glasgow: Glasgow District Libraries, 1988).

Blackmore, Susan, *The Meme Machine,* (Oxford: Oxford University Press, 1999).

Blair, Robert, *The Grave* (London: Scatcherd and Whitaker, 1747).

Bridie, James, *The Sleeping Clergyman and Other Plays* (London: Constable and Co., 1950).

Brown, George Douglas, *The House with the Green Shutters* (Edinburgh: The Mercat Press, 1986).

Brown, Dr. John, *Horae Subsecivae* (London: Adam and Charles Black, 1897).

—, *Horae Subsecivae: A Second Series* (London: Adam and Charles Black, 1897).

—, *Horae Subsecivae:Third Series* (London: Adam and Charles Black, 1897).

—, *Horae Subsecivae*, in three volumes (Series), (London: Adam and Charles Black, 1900).

Buchan, John , *Hunting Tower*, 1st pub. 1922 (London: Hamlyn Paperbacks, 1982),

—,*The House of the Four Winds*, 1st pub. 1935 (Stroud: Alan Suton, 1993)

—, *Sick Heart River,* originally published posthumously in 1941 (Harmondsworth: Penguin Books, 1985).

Burns, Robert, *The Complete Poetical Works of Robert Burns*, ed. James Mackay (Darvel: Alloway Publishing, 1993).

—, *Robert Burns' Commonplace Book*, ed. R. L. Brown (Wakefield: S and R Publishers Ltd., 1969).

Crawford, Robert and Mick Imlah, eds., *The Penguin Book of Scottish Verse,* 2nd edn., (The Penguin Press, 2000).

Cronin, A. J., *Adventures of a Black Bag* (London: New English Library, 1979).

—, *The Citadel* (London: Hodder and Stoughton, 1961).

Currie, James, *Medical Reports on the Effects of Water, Cold and Warm, as a Remedy in Fever and Febrile Diseases, Whether Applied to the Surface of the Body, or Used as a Drink, with Observations on the Nature of Fever and on the Effects of Opium, Alcohol and Inanition*, 4th edn (London: T Cadel and W Davies, 1805).

Dunbar, William, *The Poems of William Dunbar*, ed. W. M. Mackenzie, (London: Faber and Faber Ltd, 1970).

Dunn, Douglas, *Elegies* (London: Faber and Faber, 1985).

Eyre-Todd, George, *The Glasgow Poets: Their Lives and Poems* (Glasgow and Edinburgh: William Hodge and Company, 1903).

Ferguson, Ron, *Geoff* (Gartocharn: Famedram Publishers, 1979).

Fergusson, Robert, *Selected Poems*, ed. James Robertson (Edinburgh: Polygon, 2007).

Forsyth, Moira, *Tell Me Where You Are* (Ross-shire: Sandstone Press , 2010).

Galloway, Janice, *The Trick is to Keep Breathing* (London: Vintage Books, 1999).

Galt, John, *Annals of the Parish,* The World's Classics, (Oxford: Oxford University Press, 1986).

—, *The Provost* (Oxford: Oxford University Press, 1982).

Gibson, Tom, *Poems and Versifications* (Glasgow: [n.p.], 1991).

Grassic Gibbon, Lewis, *A Scots Quair: A Trilogy of Novels* (London: Hutchison, 1982).

Gray, Alasdair, *Poor things: Episodes from the Early Life of Archibald McCandless M.D., Scottish Public Health Officer* (London: Bloomsbury, 2002).

Griffin, Richard, ed., *The Letters of Robert Burns* (Glasgow: Richard Griffin and Co., 1828).

Gunn, Neil M., *The Silver Darlings* (London: Faber and Faber, 1978).

Hamilton, Walter, ed., *Poems and Parodies in Praise of Tobacco (An Odd Volume for Smokers: A Lyttlel Parcel of Poems and Parodies in Praise of Tobacco Collected by Walter Hamilton)*, (London: Reeves and Turner, 1889).

Hamilton, William of Gilbertfield, 'The Last Dying Words of Bonny Heck, a Famous Grey-hound in the Shire of Fife', in Christopher MacLachlan, ed., *Before Burns: Eighteenth-Century Scottish Poetry* (Edinburgh: Canongate Classics, 2002).

Hayward, Brian, ed., *Galoshins: The Scottish Folk Play* (Edinburgh: Edinburgh University Press, 1992).

Hogg, James, 'Elegy on the Death of a Child', in *Blackwood's Edinburgh Magazine*, 2.7 (1817), 47.

—, *The Private Memoirs and Confessions of a Justified Sinner* (London: Penguin Books, 1983).

—, 'Seeking the Houdie', in *The Devil and the Giro: Two Centuries of Scottish Stories* (Edinburgh: Canongate, 1989).

Holloway, Richard, *Leaving Alexandria* (Edinburgh: Canongate, 2012).

Hunter, John, *Works of John Hunter*, 4 vols (London: Longman, Rees, Orme, Brown, Green and Longman, 1835–1837).

Jenkins, Robin, *The Cone-Gatherers* (Edinburgh: Canongate, 2004).

Koestler, Arthur, *The Act of Creation* (London: Hutchison, 1964).

Lindsay, Maurice, *The Burns Encyclopedia* (New York: Robert Hale, 1980).

Linklater, Eric, *White-Maa's Saga* (London: Jonathan Cape, 1937).

Lochhead, Liz, *The Colour of Black and White* (Edinburgh: Polygon, 2005).

Logan, W.H., ed., *A Pedlar's Pack of Ballads and Songs* (Edinburgh: W. Paterson, 1869).

MacDiarmid, Hugh, *Complete Poems*, eds. Michael Grieve and W.R. Aitken (Manchester: Carcanet, 1993).

—, *Second Hymn to Lenin and other poems* (London: Stanley Nott, 1935)

—, *The Hugh MacDiarmid Anthology*, eds. Michael Grieve and Alexander Scott (London: Routledge and Kegan Paul, 1975).

—, *Selected Poetry,* eds. Alan Riach and Michael Grieve (Manchester, Carcanet Press, 1992).

MacDonald, Alexander, Baillie of Canna, *The Resurrection of the Ancient Scottish Language, or the New Highland Songster* (Edinburgh: [n.pub], 1751).

MacKenzie, W. Mackay, ed., *The Poems of William Dunbar* (London: Faber and Faber Ltd, 1970).

Mackenzie, Henry, *The Man of Feeling*, ed. Brian Vickers (Oxford: Oxford University Press, 1987).

Mackie, E. L., ed., *A Book of Scottish Verse* (Oxford: Oxford University Press, 1956).

MacLachlan, Christopher, ed., *Before Burns: Eighteenth-Century Scottish Poetry* (Edinburgh: Canongate Classics, 2002).

Maclaren, Ian, *Beside the Bonnie Brier Bush* (New York: Dodd, Mead and Co., 1895).

—, *A Doctor of the Old School* (La Vergne, TN: Kessinger Publishing, 2009).

McArthur, A., and H. Kingsley Long, *No Mean City* (London: Corgi Books, 1957).

McGonagall, William, *Last Poetic Gems* (Dundee: David Winter and Sons, 1971).

—, *Poetic Gems* (Dundee: David Winter and Sons, 1971).

McIlvanney, William, *Docherty* (London: Sceptre Press, 1987).

McLellen, Robert, *Sweet Largie Bay and Arran Burn: Two Poems in Scots* (Preston: Akros Publications, 1977).

McNaughton, Adam, 'Cholesterol', http://mysongbook.de/msb/songs/c/choleste.html (accessed 04/12/2013).

McSeveney, Angela, 'The Lump' in *Dream State, the New Scottish Poets*, ed. Donny O' Rouke, 2nd ed. (Edinburgh: Edinburgh University Press, 2002).

Morgan, Edwin, *A Book of Lives* (Manchester: Carcanet, 2007).

Muir, Edwin, *The Story and the Fable* (London: G.G. Harran and Co., 1940).

Murray, Prof. Robin, Personal communication.

Oliphant, Margaret, *Passages in the Life of Mrs Margaret Maitland of Sunnyside, Written by Herself* (New York: D. Appleton, 1851).

Paterson, J.R., 'Castle of Healing', in *Random Rhymes* (Clydebank: Clydebank Press, 1948).

Pittock, Murray, Personal communication, 2011.

Ramsay, Allan, 'A Poem to the Memory of Alexander Pitcairne' (1713), in *The Bibliotheck*, 7 (1979), 153–160.

—, *The Gentle Shepherd* (Edinburgh: George Reid, Printers, 1798).

—, *The Poems of Allan Ramsay*, 2 vols (Paisley: Alex Gardner, 1877).

Robertson, James, *And the Land Lay Still*, (London: Penguin Books, 2010).

Rowling, J. K., *Harry Potter and the Philosopher's Stone* (London: Bloomsbury, 1997).

Scott, Tom, ed., *The Penguin Book of Scottish Verse* (London: Penguin Books, 1970).

Scott, Walter, *Rob Roy* (Oxford: Oxford World Classics, 2008).

—, *St. Ronan's Well* (London: The Caxton Publishing Co., 1903).

—, *The Surgeon's Daughter* (London: The Caxton Publishing Company, 1903).

—, *The Talisman* (London: J.M. Dent, 1980).

Shakespeare, William, *William Shakespeare: The Collected Works*, eds. Stanley Wells, Gary Taylor, John Jowett and William Montgomery (Oxford: Clarendon Press, 1988).

Smith, Adam, *The Theory of Moral Sentiments*, eds. D.D. Raphael and A.L. Macfie (Indianapolis: Liberty Fund, 1984).

Smollett, Tobias, *The Adventures of Roderick Random*, ed. Paul-Gabriel Bouce (Oxford: Oxford University Press, 1999).

—, *The Expedition of Humphry Clinker* (Oxford: Oxford University Press, 1998).

Soutar, William, *Diaries of a Dying Man*, ed. Alexander Scott (Edinburgh: W & R Chambers, 1954).

Stevenson, Robert Louis, *A Child's Garden of Verse* (London: Longmans Green and Co., 1926).

—, *Kidnapped* (Edinburgh: Polygon, 2007).

—, *The Strange Case of Dr Jekyll and Mr Hyde* (London: William Heinemann, 1924).

—, *Treasure Island* (London: Cassell and Company, 1950).

—, *Underwoods and Ballads* (Charleston: Bibliobazaar, 2006).

—, *Weir of Hermiston* (London: Penguin Books, 1979).

Thomson, James (B.V.), *The City of Dreadful Night* (Glasgow: Kennedy and Boyd, 2008).

Todd, Margaret, *Mona Maclean, Medical Student* (London and Glasgow: Collins Clear Type Press, 1892).

Wallace, William, ed., *Robert Burns and Mrs Dunlop: Correspondence Now Published in Full* (London: Hodder and Stoughton, 1898).

Welsh, Irvine, *Trainspotting* (London: Minerva, 1996).

Whistle-Binkie: A Collection of Songs for the Social Circle (Glasgow: David Robertson, 1846).

Whyte, Hamish, ed., *Mungo's Tongues: Glasgow Poems 1630–1990* (Edinburgh: Mainstream Publishing, 1993).

Wiseman, Richard, *Severall Chirurgical Treatises* (London: [n. pub.], 1676).

Secondary Sources

Bacon, Francis, *The Advancement of Learning, Novum Organum, New Atlantis*, I (Chicago: William Benton, 1952).

Banks, Ian, *The Wasp Factory* (London: Macmillan, 1984).

Bannerman, John, *The Beatons, a Medical Kindred in the Classical Gaelic Tradition.* (Edinburgh: John Donald Publishers Ltd, 1998).

Barbour, John, *The Bruce,* ed. and trans, A.A.M. Duncan, (Edinburgh: Cannongate Classics, 1997).

Bayliss, J.H., 'Epidemiological Considerations of the History of Indigenous Malaria in Britain', *Endeavour*, 9 (1985), 191–94.

Beatson, Sir George, 'On the Treatment of Incurable Cancer of the Mamma: Suggestions of a New Method of Treatment', *The Lancet*, 2 (1896), 104–7.

Blackwell, Elizabeth, *Pioneering Work in Opening the Medical Profession to Women* (London: Longmans Green and Co, 1895).

Blind Harry, *Wallace*, rev. William Hamilton of Gilbertfield (Edinburgh: Luath Press, 1996).

Bolton, Gillie, *The Therapeutic Potential of Creative Writing* (London and Philadelphia: Jessica Kingsley Publisher, 1999).

Brockington, C.F., *Public Health in the 19th Century* (Edinburgh: E and S Livingstone, 1965).

Buchan, William, *Buchan's Domestic Medicine, or a Treatise on the Prevention and Cure of Disease by Regimen and Simple Medicines* (Edinburgh: Arch Allardice, 1824).

Budd, Adam, *John Armstrong's The Art of Preserving Health* (Farnham: Ashgate, 2011).

Building Up on our Health: The Architecture of Scotland's Historic Hospitals ([n.p.]: Historic Scotland, 2010).

Bymun, W.F., and R. Porter, *Companion Encyclopaedia of the History of Medicine* (London and New York: Routledge, 1993).

Caldwell, Janis McLaren, *Literature and Medicine in Nineteenth-Century Britain: From Mary Shelley to George Eliot* (Cambridge: Cambridge University Press, 2004).

Calman, K.C., *A Study of Storytelling, Humour and Learning in Medicine* (London: The Stationery Office, 2000).

—, *Medical Education: Past, Present and Future* (Edinburgh: Elsevier, 2007).

—, *The Potential for Health* (Oxford: Oxford University Press, 1998).

—, 'The Profession of Medicine', *British Medical Journal*, (1994), 1140–3.

—, 'Quality of Life in Cancer Patients', *Journal of Medical Ethics*, 228 (1984), 585–87.

—, and R.S. Downie, 'Why Arts Courses for Medicine?', *Lancet*, (1996), 1499–50.

—, R.S. Downie, M. Duthie, B. Sweeney, 'Literature and Medicine: A Course', *Medical Education*, 22 (1988), 265–69.

Cameron, James K., *The First Book of Discipline: with Introduction and Commentary* (Edinburgh: Saint Andrew Press, 1972).

Campbell, J.L., *Canna: The Story of a Hebridean Island*, 3rd ed. (Oxford: Oxford University Press, 1994).

Carnegie, Andrew, *The Gospel of Wealth and Other Timely Essays*, 3rd ed. (London: Frederick Warne, 1903).

Chalmers, A.K., *The Health of Glasgow 1818–1925: An Outline* (Glasgow: Corporation of Glasgow, 1930).

—, *Public Health Administration in Glasgow: a Memorial Volume of the Writings of James Burn Russell* (Glasgow: James Maclehose and Sons, 1905).

Chalmers, Thomas, *Problems of Poverty: An Enquiry into the Industrial Condition of the Poor* (London: Thomas Nelson and Sons, 1912).

Chambers, R., *The Traditions of Edinburgh* (Edinburgh: W.R Chambers, 1868).

Chin, T., and P.D. Welsby, 'Malaria in the UK: Past, Present and Future', *Postgraduate Medical Journal*, 80 (2004), 663–666.

Clift, Stephen, 'Creative Arts as a Public Health Resource: Moving from Practice-based Research to Evidence-based Practice', *Perspectives in Public Health*, 132 (2012), 120–127.

Cluness, A.T., article in *The Scotsman*, 1962, from a typed transcript.

Comrie, J.D., *History of Scottish Medicine* in Two Volumes (London: Bailliere, Tindall and Cox, 1932).

Daiches, David, *Robert Fergusson* (Edinburgh: Scottish Academic Press, 1982).

Dingwall, H., D. Hamilton, I. Macintyre, M. McCrae, D. Wright, *Scottish Medicine: An Illustrated History* (Edinburgh: Birlinn, 2011).

Dobson, M. J., 'History of Malaria in England', *Journal of the Royal Society of Medicine*, 82 (1989), 3–7.

Duncan, K., and Proc.R.Coll, 'The Possible Influence of Climate Change on Historical Outbreaks of Malaria in Scotland', *Physicians Edinb.*, 23 (1993), 55–62.

Ferguson, Adam, *Essay on the History of Civil Society*, ed. Fania Oz-Salzberger (London: Transaction Publications, 1995).

Findlay, William, *Robert Burns and the Medical Profession* (London: Alexander Gardiner, 1898).

Flynn, Michael, ed., *Scottish Population History from the 17th Century to the 1930s* (Cambridge: Cambridge University Press, 1977).

Friedson, E., 'The Limits of Professional Autonomy', in *Profession of Medicine* (New York: Dodd, Mead and Company, 1975).

Gairdner, Sir William Tennant, *The Physician as Naturalist* (Glasgow: James Maclehose, 1889).

Gillies, H. Cameron, *Regimen Sanitatis. From the Vade Mecum of the Famous Mac-Beaths, Physicians to the Lords of the Isles and the Kings of Scotland for Several Centuries* (Glasgow: Alex MacLaren and Sons, 1911).

Grant, Ted, and Sandy Carter, *Women in Medicine: A Celebration of Their Work* (Ontario: Firefly Books, 2004).

Grosart, Alexander, *Robert Fergusson* (Edinburgh: Oliphant, Anderson and Ferrier, 1898).

Gull, S.E., R. O'Flynn, and J.Y.L. Hunter, 'Creative Writing Workshops for Medical Education', *Medical Humanities*, 28 (2002), 102–4.

Hamilton, D., *The Healers: A History of Medicine in Scotland* (Edinburgh: Cannongate, 1981).

Haraldsottir, E., 'Poetry and Creative Writing in Palliative Care', *British Medical Journal*, Supportive and Palliative Care, 1 (2011), 260.

Henryson, Robert. *Poems and Fables*, eds. H. Harvery Wood and James Thin (Edinburgh: Mercat Press, 1933).

Hippocrates, 'Aphorism 1', in *The Genuine Works of Hippocrates*, trans. Francis Adams (Baltimore: William and Wilkins, 1939).

Holmes, Oliver Wendell, *The Professor at the Breakfast Table* (London: Routledge, 1905).

Hume, Ruth Fox, *Great Women in Medicine* (New York: Random House, 1964).

Hunter, D., and R.R. Romford, *Hutchison's Clinical Methods*, 13th ed (London: Cassell, 1956).

Hurd-Mead, Kate Campbell, *A History of Women in Medicine* (New York: AMS Press, 1977).

Johnston, Thomas, *History of the Working Classes in Scotland* (Glasgow: Forward, 1929).

Katzev, R.D., *In the Country of Books: Commonplace Books and Other Readings* (Matador, Leicester, 2009).

Maureen Kerr, *George Murray, A School Teacher for St Kilda* (Islands Book Trust, 2013).

Kyd, J.G., (ed.), 'Scottish Population History from the 17th Century to the 1930s', in *Scottish Population Statistics (third series)* (Edinburgh: Scottish History Society, 1952), XL III.

Leask, Nigel, 'Robert Burns and the Stimulant Regime' in *Fickle Man: Robert Burns in the 21st century*, eds. J.Rodger and G. Carruthers (Ross-shire: Sandstone Press, 2009).

Lindsay, Sir David, *A Satire of the Three Estates*, adapted for Tyrone Guthrie's production at the 1948 Edinburgh Festival. Introduction and notes by Matthew McDiarmid (London: Heinmann Educational Books, 1967).

MacKenzie, John, *Sar-obair nam Bard Gaelach*. 4th ed. trans. Hugh Cheape (Edinburgh: 1877) pp. 389–90.

Martin, Martin, *A Description of the Western Isles of Scotland* (Edinburgh: Birlinn Press, 1999).

Morgan, Edward, 'A Scottish Trawl', in Christopher Whyte, *Gendering the Nation: Studies in Modern Scottish Literature* (Edinburgh: Edinburgh University Press, 1995).

Morgan, Nicola, *Fleshmarket,* (London: Hodder Children's Books, 2003).

Morris, Ruth and Frank, *Scottish Healing Wells* (Sandy: The Alethea Press, 1982).

Moss, Ann, *Printed Commonplace Books* (Oxford: Oxford University Press, 1996).

Murray, James A.H. ed., *The Complaynt of Scotland*, 1st pub 1872 (Wales: Llanerch Publishers, reprint 1998).

Nash, Andrew, *Kailyard and Scottish Literature* (Amsterdam: Rodopi, 2001).

O'Mahony, S., 'A.J. Cronin and *The Citadel*: did a work of fiction contribute to the foundation of the NHS?', *J.R.Coll. Physicians*, 42 (2012), 172–8.

Office for National Statistics. *Lifestyle Survey Overview. A Report of the 2010 General Lifestyle Survey* (Newport: National Statistics Publication, 2012).

Osler, William, *Aequanimitas, With Other Addresses* (London: H.K. Lewis, 1904).

—, *The Principles and Practice of Medicine*, 9th ed. (New York: B. Appleton and Co., 1921).

—, *The Student Life: The Philosophy of William Osler*, ed. R.E. Verney (Edinburgh: E and S Livingstone, 1957).

The Oxford Dictionary of Quotations, 3rd ed. (Oxford: Oxford University Press, 1980).

Paton, D.N., J.C. Dunlop, and E. Inglis, *A Study of the Diet of the Laboring Classes in Edinburgh* (Edinburgh: Otto Schulte and Company, 1906).

Roy, J., 'Malaria in England Past, Present and Future', *Soc. Promotion of Health*, 94 (1974), 23–29.

Scott, Thomas Bodley, Obituary, *British Medical Journal*, 1 (1924), 297–8.

Smith, G. Gregory, *Scottish Literature: Character and Influence* (London: MacMillan and Co., 1919).

Smout, T.C., *A Century of the Scottish People 1830-1950* (London: Fontana Press, 1986).

Sutherland, John, 'Stories for Boys', *Times Literary Supplement*, 18 November 2011.

Tait, H.P., *A Doctor and Two Policemen: The History of the Edinburgh Health Department* (Edinburgh: Mackenzie and Storie, 1974).

Thornton, Robert Donald, *William Maxwell to Robert Burns* (Edinburgh: John Donald Publishers, 1979).

Tournier, Paul, *Creative Suffering* (San Francisco: Harper Row Publishing, 1983).

Watson, Roderick, *The Literature of Scotland: Middle Ages to the Nineteenth Century* (NewYork, N.Y: Palgrave MacMillan, 2007).

World Health Organisation., Preamble to the Constitution of the World Health Organisation, *Official Records of World Health Organisation,* 10 (1946).

—, Symposium, *The pen is as mighty as the Surgeon's Scalpel,* WHO Regional Office 1988

Yeats, L.A., Letter, *Times Literary Supplement*, 25 November 2011, p. 6.

Index

Headings in *italic* are titles of literary works noted in the text